A Year with Misty

Manders Smith

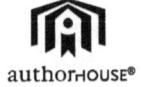

authorHOUSE®

AuthorHouse™ UK Ltd.
500 Avebury Boulevard
Central Milton Keynes, MK9 2BE
www.authorhouse.co.uk
Phone: 08001974150

First published by AuthorHouse 8/14/2009

ISBN: 978-1-4490-0747-8 (sc)

This book is printed on acid-free paper.

Once upon a time…

Well it's a fairy story as it's about a couple of old Queens. But also true.

So what is it?

A tale of sexual tranny depravity!

Well, no, actually it's not. It's nothing shocking, and certainly there's nothing overtly erotic or sexual in it.

If you were seeking something like that, then you are reading the wrong book.

Okay, well, there is a reference to sex, but more by way of innuendo, and no graphic details!

Essentially it's a journey of discovery from sex to true love - tranny love.

Sex is what drives trannies, and I had the battle scars to prove it! But sex was not what I really wanted, and in truth neither do most trannies if we're honest.

We all want love!

Misty showed me that even gurlz like us could fall in love!

A rare thing in the transitory TV world!

Before I met Misty my life was in utter and total confusion!

It's one thing not knowing where you're going, but things get even trickier when you can't find the captain who's supposed to be flying the bloody plane.

In my case I couldn't make my mind up whether I was the pilot or some trolley dolly who was halfway down the aisle looking for the nearest parachute.

It ain't easy being a bloke and a gurl at the same time!

Shortly after meeting Misty I started keeping a diary of everything that happened between us.

I don't really know why, because I've never kept a diary in my entire life, so this was something of a novelty for me.

Maybe it was because I sensed something, and would soon find out she was ill.

Partly I wanted to be able to recollect the events, but I prefer to think it was because we had something very special in our lives, and I wanted to be able to remember it all just the way it happened.

Mainly it's about my times with Misty. It was a rocky road with lots of highs and lows. I know we found a love that transcended sex and that in itself was worth recording.

I wasn't sure what I was going to do with the diary, but I thought I might give it to Misty as a special present when we reached our first anniversary.

It would be a nice reminder to us both of the times we spent together and she could read it while she recuperated.

Well, it wasn't to be.

Life is fragile!

I guess for all of us gurlz dressing is not something we chose to do.

It's not an illness either.

It's just there, and when it's there all you can do is make the best of a bad job, which is what Misty and I did.

<u>Saturday 7 April 2007</u>

I was contracting down in Aylesbury on my fourth contract and used to come home to Sleaford, in Lincolnshire, at weekends.

That's when Misty first contacted me on a well-known transvestite dating site.

tvChix

The site has various chat rooms where TVs can meet other TVs, or admirers, or even RGs (Real Girls) if they're so inclined.

Before we go any further I ought to explain a bit of terminology so you know what is what in our world!

Gender-bending stuff!

Admirers are men who date TVs as women. Most are married and generally regard TVs as fair game for extra curricular activities. They tend to be notoriously unreliable.

The life of a TV!

Then there are partners of TVs who either tolerate or join in the lifestyle to some degree or another. For some it works okay, but for others it is the beginning of divorce proceedings.

Risky business!

There are HPWs, who in longhand are known as Hairy Panty Wearers (or cross-dressers).

How most of us start out!

These are guys who wear their own or their wives' lingerie. A few meet, but for the majority it's a secret thing they do when the wife's out.

For most it's just a fetish that gives them some form of sexual excitement!

Also, the site is not restricted to men and their partners.

You might be surprised at the number of RGs there in their own right.

They are not partners of anyone else but just seem to enjoy the company of TVs (usually called associates).

Then there are the gurlz who have had some modification done around their chests but still retain their male genitalia.

Boobies!

Suppose they can be called pre-op gurlz.

They should not be confused with true transsexuals, who have had most of their physical male aspects stripped away and are now ostensibly changed into womanhood.

Post-op gurlz!

They tend to be very touchy about the way they are referred to or labelled. Many describe themselves as women who had transsexual pasts before they fully transitioned.

I'm not sure if I've ever worked that one out!

I always thought they were males of some description, at least in body, before they transitioned.

I know I'll get my wrists slapped for saying that, but until they invent a male womb, that's my version!

I suppose to complete the suite I ought to mention the very small percentage of those called intersexed, or what you may know as hermaphrodites.

Yes, they do exist!

Most of the members of tvChix are just common or garden-variety TVs.

Like me, I guess!

Some TVs are gay, some are bi, and a few say they are straight.

Not sure I'm convinced about the "straight" ones!

When you join the site you can set up a profile for yourself. It describes what you are:

HPWs, TV, pre-op transsexual, post-op transsexual, admirer, or associate.

"Pre-op transsexual" is a much misused term. A lot of TVs seem to think it gives them some special standing in the community!

What a load of old twaddle!

You either going for the chop or you're not.

And then you can add pictures of yourself if you want to let people know what you look like.

Helps if yours are current!

There are a lot of phoney ones on there and loads that are miles out of date.

There are in truth a lot of dreamers and fantasists on this site, and it's not till you've been on there a while that you get a sixth sense of who you're talking to.

The question of what people put in their profiles is another good indication of who you might be dealing with.

Some are short and to the point, some have humour, and some are endless diatribes which go on forever.

Usually the long ones are composed of some self-inflicted angst which people seem to think has some deep meaning to others.

More twaddle!

Anyway, back to Misty.

She obviously liked my profile and my pictures, and she left a couple of messages which I replied to. One thing led to another and soon we started talking on the phone on a regular basis.

I called her Misty because that's the name she liked to be called in person, although on the website her profile was Oz Michelle.

As you can tell from the "Oz", she was an Australian gurl.

Normally she rang me when I went shopping on Saturday mornings at the local Tesco. I remember sitting in the car park chatting endlessly to her. Very easy to talk with.

I can't really remember too much of what we talked about, except that she was in the process of closing a deal.

She had been out of work for a while and was buying a business. We were trying to fit that around me meeting her at her cottage in London.

Initially the plan was for me to go down and stay over one night while I was contracting in Aylesbury.

She reckoned it was only about forty minutes away, so I could get back to Aylesbury in the morning for work.

We arranged a date, but unfortunately she had to cancel it at the last minute. Something cropped up over the business she was buying. Anyway, we put it on hold.

How many times had I heard that before!

I thought it would be the usual story and peter out into nothing, as so many potential meets do.

Anyway, we kept in contact, and the one thing I really remember is the way she talked.

Mmm!

She still had a slight Australian twang and a lovely husky drawling voice.

Very "come to bed"!

It seemed so warm and caring despite her really outrageous pictures on the site. The one thing that really struck me was that underneath it all she seemed so normal!

A few weeks later my contract ended, so I was back in Sleaford.

One Friday evening I was on Yahoo! and the website in the evening, just looking to see what was about. I wasn't looking to sort anything out in terms of a meeting, as I had one arranged. I was just chatting to so-called "friends".

That's another term I use in inverted commas, because the word friend is such a misused word in our world. I've spoken to so many gurlz over the years that have what they call a wide circle of friends!

FFS (for f… sake)!

It's all based on dressing up and whatever other activity goes on. It's not real.

True friendship only comes when gurlz can strip all the female pretence away.

I often laugh when I see pictures of gurlz together which have a label at the bottom that says something like:

"Me and my best gurl at such and such an event"

You know full well that they probably only met once or twice. You wonder what they'd be like as man on man when all the gurly stuff has gone.

Anyway, Misty asked me on Yahoo! if I could meet her on the Saturday, but initially I told her I couldn't, as I'd arranged to go and see Debbie down in Hemel Hempstead.

Debbie was a gurl I'd already seen a couple of times while I was in Aylesbury. When I heard the contract had ended, we'd arranged for me to go and see her again and for me to stop overnight.

She was okay when dressed, but *en* drab she was really intense and used to get worked up about the smallest of things.

It drove me to distraction, and I knew it would never last.

We had nothing in common, and the only reason I had been to see her a few times was because we'd worked out a good role play between us.

Kinky bedroom games!

It was always a fantasy of mine to enact certain scenes with a partner, and with most people you never get the opportunity. Everything is too rushed.

As part of the preparation I brought a maid's outfit from another website and had it delivered to Debbie's flat.

It was good quality, not a cheap tatty dress like you can buy from most sites. The dress itself was black, came down to about knee length, and had a zip in the side so it fitted snugly round the waist.

The bust area and the sleeves were finished off with ruffled white material with frilly ends, so it all trimmed the whole tunic off nicely.

When I ordered it I bought a couple of little flounced petticoats to go with it. They really filled the skirt out, and the whole outfit was tied off at the waist with a little frilly white apron.

I even got a frilly pink suspender belt to go with it all, and as a final touch there was a little ornamental flower which I stuck in my wig.

Almost looked like a genuine French maid.

Ooh la la - well, a camp one!

Once I was fully dressed she used to take me to her brass bed. All rods and such.

Without going into detail, let's just say she was well practised in her knotting technique, and the maid's outfit seemed to do the trick. I was the naughty maid!

Anyway Misty wasn't taking no for an answer, and she rang me. She said she wanted to see me on the Saturday, as she'd just closed her big business deal and would really like me to come down and help her celebrate.

She was extremely persuasive, and somehow I thought we might have more in common than I had with Debbie.

I always remember the phrase she used which finally swung it for me.

"You've tried the rest; now try the best."

Well, gullible and excited me couldn't refuse such a beguiling offer, and I agreed.

I'd spent ages thinking up a good story as an excuse for not seeing Debbie. We're all so fickle, so coming up with something plausible was not unusual.

I'm not sure what happened to Debbie, as she seems to have disappeared from the scene altogether. I just hope I wasn't partly responsible for that.

We're all very much like moths that get drawn towards the brightest light.

Misty had it in spades at the time!

I remember asking her if she had a spare room for me to sleep in that night. Not because I wanted to. I just didn't fancy ending up sleeping on a couch.

She told me not to worry as she'd take care of me, so I just said okay. When we spoke about it at a later date she said my question had sounded really strange.

Thought she'd got hold of a right one that night!

Misty emailed me the directions, and I arranged to go down on Saturday afternoon and arrive at about five.

I had an eighteen-year-old son at home, but he was quite glad to be rid of me so he could spend some time alone with his girlfriend.

Think he was glad to see the back of the old poof!

I was dreading driving down to London. But from what Misty said she was right on the northern outskirts, so I wouldn't have to actually drive through London itself, which was a blessed relief.

Cricklewood, here I come!

It didn't take too long to get there but towards the end of the M1 I took the turning off to Brentwood instead of going to the end, as Misty had told me to do.

Doh! - Got lost as usual!

I had to ring her a couple of times for further directions and must admit I had such a fear of London that I almost got to the point of driving home. From Brentwood it must have taken me almost a half hour to find the right road into London, which Misty said would take me right to her house.

I still had to drive about three miles though Cricklewood, but eventually I found her turnoff on the left, and it was a huge relief to be pulling off the main drag.

In the email she had told me to park the car in a little side street and then go to her house and pick up parking permits.

When I found her house and knocked on the door she opened it very slightly, and this hand appeared with two tickets.

I noticed she had beautifully painted nails and rings on.

Fully dressed for my arrival!

I put the tickets on the car and grabbed my suitcase from the boot. When I got back the door was still slightly ajar, as Misty had said it would be.

Misty was nowhere to be seen, which was exactly as she said it would be in her mail.

I had already sent her a picture of me *en* drab so she'd know what to expect.

She said in earlier conversations that she didn't need to know any details about the drab me, and she certainly didn't want to see the drab me when I arrived. I did think it a little bit shallow - so just the usual TV meet.

Sex was on the menu - no surprises, then!

The back door opened into the kitchen, and I went straight through that and into to the lounge, which had curtains drawn and some lights on in preparation.

It was still light outside and the lounge window looked straight into the house across the road. Misty didn't want to make it too obvious to her neighbours.

Mind you it was more about people walking past the widow, than the neighbours opposite.

Some very nice former police ladies lived together there!

At the far side of the lounge on the left there was another door, which led to the stairs and the upstairs rooms.

As instructed I heaved my case up the steep stairs and plonked it in the bathroom.

I closed the door and could hear Misty in the room next door, so I shouted and asked if I could have a bath. She said that was fine.

Bathing is a tranny ritual!

Must have taken me about an hour or so to have a bath and get dressed and do my makeup.

Won't bore you with the details, but I wore my black girdle with suspenders and a strapless bra, as I was going to wear my halter-neck black and white print dress.

I made sure I had plenty of stockings in case I laddered any and strappy black sandals with 5-inch heels.

At that time I had a short auburn wig and big round clip-on earrings, plus a fake gemstone choker. When I was totally ready I sprayed myself with body spray and perfume, which at the time was Poison.

Can't be a proper gurly if you don't smell right!

I must admit I was slightly nervous as I teetered down the stairs in my heels with a bottle of wine in one hand and the other clutching the rail.

Always took wine on a first date - another tranny ritual.

But I do remember that as I entered the lounge we both smiled at each other, and something told me it was going to be okay between us that night.

From a transvestite's point of view I thought Misty looked superb.

TVs have a different perspective on beauty!

She was quite tall, as a lot of TVs tend to be, very slender, and looked very slinky in her outfit.

Two sofas were on either side of the coffee table, so to start with I sat on the one opposite her, by the window.

Well, you have to go through the niceties!

Behind my sofa was a small modern dresser with flowers on it and her cat, called Eddy.   He was asleep on it, oblivious to what we were doing or going to do.

The lights were down nice and low, and there was the sound of Massachusetts coming from the stereo in the form of George Thoroghgood and the Destroyers live.

Seemed to set the scene.

Misty poured some wine for us both. We did the usual chitchat about previous experiences which always helps break the ice.

We discovered we had a "friend" in common, Angie. I'd seen her a couple of times. With me it was just "poppers", but by the time she came to see Misty she'd graduated to coke. Often the way with a lot of TVs. Drugs seem to be part of the culture.

Bad news!

I was a bit awestruck with Misty and remember I even mentioned in passing that I used to escort a bit.

I had hoped that might impress her a little and make me seem like I'd been around a bit.

Which I had - think I was due for an oil change!

Misty talked about a few things she'd done in the past. She seemed like a worldly gurl who'd definitely been round the block a few times more than me.

LOL (laughed out loud) - two old troopers together!

She told me she had a sub slut in training called Sabrina, which sounded impressive.

Well it did to a little country gurl like me.

She'd recently had Sabrina tied to the table in front of us as part of her training and forgotten how tight she'd tied her. She begged to be released, and Misty told me she just kept her there, as she hadn't noticed what pain she was in. It was all said in humour and we laughed at that.

At that stage I thought she was really an accomplished dom. She seemed to have it all in terms of confidence and poise.

I got the impression she'd really played the field and I would end up as just another notch on her bedpost. Oh well!

We chatted for a while, and it wasn't long before Misty went to get another bottle of wine.

I was feeling a bit braver by then, and when she came back she found me sitting on the same sofa as her. I guess that was the only signal she needed, and it all started to get very touchy-feely.

We both eased towards each other until one thing led to another, and we ended up kissing and cuddling.

Usual stuff - but very nice!

Sex did play a part in the evening.

No surprises there then!

But there was something more going on then. There was
a feeling in the air.

Most of it was just cuddling together and sharing those
things that you can never really confide in others outside
of the TV world.

Just felt so right - everything clicked.

I guess that's one of the reasons neither of us realised what
the time was, as we just wanted it to go on and on.

As the sun chinked through the curtains in the early
morning it must have been getting on for nearly five.

I remember that as we chatted about meeting other gurlz
I said one thing which misty reminded me of some time
later.

I said that gurlz don't meet and get attached. It's all very
transitory.

What a lie that was - she had already captured my heart.

There was a lot of bravado going on with me then!

I kidded myself that it was just another meeting for sex
and would end up as nothing more.

I know we'd only met once, but in truth it was like nothing I'd ever known before.

It just seemed we had simpatico from the start and everything else just fell into place.

I told you I'd been round the block, and just to give you some idea, I'd met about 200 gurlz and guyz before this.

Qualified trollop of the first degree!

This wasn't a new experience to me, but as the evening wore on, I suddenly found all my usual feelings of being an experienced gurl being swept aside.

I found myself feeling very small and inexperienced by all this. I know I didn't show it on the outside, but inside I was feeling very vulnerable with all my defences down.

I always thought I was beyond all this!

Okay, there had been some slight pangs in the past when meeting other gurlz, but nothing quite like this.

Felt I was totally out of my depth, like a drowning gurl who had suddenly had a lifebelt thrown to her.

Could there really be more to this, and did I have some chance of grasping it?

I knew it was only a fanciful whim, so I put it to the back of my mind. I just thought that one day I'd look back on all this and say what if it had been?

That would be nice rosy thing to fantasise about in the future.

Later that night, or should I say early in the morning, Misty made some coffee and asked me if I'd like a regular or espresso.

I always loved the way she made espresso, and that became my drink. She used to make some for me each time I arrived at her house.

Misty had her usual coffee, which was a regular coffee with two sugars, and half of it was made from condensed cream.

She brought them all in on a tray with little amaretto biscuits.

Just seemed so civilised.

She poured us each a large whisky in lovely crystal-cut tumblers.

Misty smoked some grass as well.

Wasn't too long before I cuddled up to Misty and desperately tried not to yawn. I just didn't want to go to bed.

Knew it would all be gone in the morning!

But I couldn't hold it off much longer, and I was just so tired as it was nearly seven in the morning.

She was in the same state as me, and eventually we both had to cave in.

Sleep was about to overtake us!

Reluctantly we both went upstairs, and Misty took me to her large double bed, as she had always intended to. Neither of us bothered removing much except our shoes and dresses. I remember almost pouring myself in between those welcoming sheets.

It wasn't the first time I had slept with a gurl. There'd been other times.

But that was all about the excitement of dressing and pretending we were gurlz.

Strange, but at the time I had felt that was exciting, but it was nothing like this.

With Misty it was different. This didn't seem like a fantasy.

All those base instincts that normally drive us on seemed to fade into insignificance.

This just felt very right and different in a way.

I don't know if it was the booze or the fact that I was so tired, but when I climbed into that bed it was like being beside someone I'd known all my life.

I was halfway asleep when Misty climbed in beside me, and I remember that warm feeling as she turned towards my back and wrapped her arms around me.

I felt like I was home for the first time in my life!

Sounds very mushy, I know, but I just drifted off as soft clouds folded over me and washed all my cares away in Misty's embrace. Nothing else seemed to matter.

I wasn't even thinking of the following morning then, but that night it felt like love was in the air.

Believe it or not, I was so full of energy that I got up early on the Sunday morning.

Well, when I say early, it was about 11.30.

I got washed and changed, packed my bag and was ready to go home.

Misty had seen a picture of me *en* drab before, as I had sent her a picture before we met, so it was no shock to her when I came down in the morning as a little bald bloke.

She was still dressed and made some coffee, which I had quickly before departing. I said thanks for the Saturday night and then said goodbye to her as you normally do.

There was no outward sign of any emotion in either of us.

She saw me to the door, and I took my suitcase and shook her hand as I left.

All very businesslike.

I really wanted to give her a kiss, but last night was gone now, and we were back in the real world.

Stupid dreaming tranny with my world about to come crashing down!

I knew I was playing with fire!

I drove back feeling so alive. It might sound corny, but I literally felt like I was floating on air.

I couldn't believe how much my sordid little world had changed in one night.

It was beyond anything I had dreamed or imagined possible.

But being a realist, I knew it was only an illusion, and I was prepared to come down to earth with a big bump.

Some things are too good to be true!

I wasn't working at the time, so I tried to put it out of my mind. I decided I had to find a new contract the next week in order to earn some pennies.

That was my mission and something to keep me occupied.

Hopefully I'd forget about Misty and it would all fade slowly away.

After all, I had no idea what she really felt about me, and I knew it wouldn't go anywhere.

They never do!

Last night was all tranny talk!

We lived too far apart to make it work.

Besides, she lived in different world than I did. It was just another TV meeting based around animal instincts and nothing more. Not a good idea to confuse Sex and Love.

Much as I tried to put it out of my mind, as I drove back, I did nothing but think of her.

Despite what I knew to be the cold truth I had a little beacon of hope inside and was just praying and hoping she'd ring or come onto Yahoo! next week and maybe we could arrange another meeting. It really did feel like being at home and I guess I was hooked.

Well, hope grows eternal, as they say!

Got home at about 2.30 and had mixed emotions. One half of me was absolutely shattered, while the other half was walking on air.

Well, the bump came!

I just sat there in the lounge and thought what a stupid sod I am!

It was just a big dream, so what do I do now?

Meeting other people now seemed pretty tawdry in comparison. The drive wasn't there anymore. I guess I had been spoilt.

My son came downstairs to the lounge and mumbled hello (as he felt obliged to) before shooting off back upstairs to see his girlfriend. When he'd gone I just sat there and felt like crying.

One night and one meeting like so many others, but this one had left me with a huge nagging pit in my stomach. I wanted to ring or text Misty but just thought that would look so stupid and naive.

I felt like a complete mess.

Didn't want to be by myself anymore.

She'd stuck a knife right in me and twisted it hard.

Wish I hadn't been there now - should have stayed in Lincs!

Thought I ought to see what messages I had on my computer. It would be the usual stuff from people I'd never met wanting a meeting for sex.

I know I had a vain hope there might be something there from Misty, but in reality I didn't think there would be.

I opened up Yahoo! and saw there was one new message, so I thought I ought to take a look and see what it was.

There was a message from Misty, but she'd sent it from her male address. It was entitled:

"Concern"!

That stopped my heart!

I suddenly felt a little sweaty shiver run down my back as the pit in my stomach opened up.

FFS!

I felt like screaming out loud!

I knew what was coming now!

"Dear John"!

Story of my life!

I clicked on the message, and I saw it started with my male name. I knew what the rest would say!

Thanks, but no thanks!

Well, she had her sophisticated life in London and knew all these gurlz and was out and about, so I just couldn't see what she wanted with a small town gurl like me.

Then I read the whole thing, which was written exactly as follows:

Hello…

I am a little concerned that Misty may be, or already has, fallen for Mandy in a big way…!

Would appreciate your advice as to whether I should intervene, talk some sense into her, or just let it go and see what happens.

Would appreciate your ideas.

With best personal regards,

M—

I couldn't believe it and read it several times.

Well, you can guess I had a warm glow all over me now!

Took ages to think up the right reply. Guess I threw caution to the wind and thought I might as well go in with both guns blazing.

Always have my heart on my sleeve!

Hello M—,

Thank you for your message regarding Manders, and your sensibility for writing to me for my advice on the subject.

Unfortunately, as you might appreciate, I can't get much sense out of her in her current lovesick state of mind, for which I hold you responsible.

I've told her over and over again that she needs to be careful and she'll only end up getting hurt if she carries on like this, but you know Manders.

Hopelessly romantic and loyal when the right person comes along.

She even told me she's more than happy for you to play with whoever you want, as she doesn't want you to be alone.

Well, if you want my advice I'd let it go and enjoy it while it's there and you feel the same way, as I know she does.

One thing I would ask, given that Manders is so soft, is just tell her when it's over.

She came back here today and was very down with it.

Do give my regards to Misty

All the best

B—

I guess Misty did feel something for me, and it might not just be tranny talk.

Hopefully at the very least it might mean another meeting was on the cards, although neither of us specifically mentioned it.

The Tuesday after the Sunday she suddenly pinged me on Yahoo!.

We started chatting, and much as I wanted to ask her if she wanted to meet again, I held back and avoided the subject. I didn't want to seem too eager!

Not too sure what we talked about, but I know the conversation went on for a while. I knew we were reaching the end, and nothing about a further meeting had been said.

Had a few collywobbles then!

Suddenly she just slipped it into the conversation and asked me casually if I was coming at the weekend.

When I heard that my heart jumped a beat. I said okay in what I hoped was a matter-of- fact way, although it's hard to get any inflection on Yahoo!.

I just didn't want to seem too desperate.

As I wasn't working, Misty suggested I went down on Friday and we could both go to BNO together.

That was quite exciting, as I'd only been to the venue where it was held once, on New Year's Eve, but had never been to an actual BNO night.

I always promised myself I'd go one day. BNO stands for the:

Big Night Out

It's held on the second Friday of every month in Pink Punters in Milton Keynes.

As the venue name might suggest, it's one the best gay clubs in Britain, and on a BNO night there's always a big gathering of TVs and admirers from tvChix.

I'd spent a lot of time in the chat rooms previously and heard a lot about it from other gurlz who'd been there. They always hyped it up and said how great it was.

At that time I thought it was the in place to go if you wanted to be accepted as part of the tranny crowd. Well, that's the sort of impression they gave me, and if you hadn't been before you didn't know any different.

Bit of a poser place - but still a great night out.

During the rest of the week we chatted most nights about all sorts of things that weren't really of any consequence.

We were still dancing around what was really happening, and neither of us mentioned anything about how we felt about each other.

You just don't normally do that in TV relationships. Well, certainly not in the early days.

I think we both kept a little distance just in case we'd been picking up the wrong signals or misinterpreting what was going on.

It's so easy to do in the fragile tranny world!

Could have been infatuation on both sides for all we knew.

<u>Friday 13 April</u>
I drove down to Misty's late on Friday afternoon and parked the car in a side street just up from Misty's house, as I had done last week.

Misty said we were still going to BNO tonight if that was okay with me.

Well, of course it was, so I went upstairs and had a bath and got changed. I wore the same things as last week, as I really didn't have a lot of other clothes for going out.

I guess most of what I had was frilly lingerie and bedroom wear, which tells you something about how I used to spend most of my time before I met Misty.

Bedroom gurl - LOL!

I know a lot of gurlz can think of nothing better than dressing up to go out, but I have always preferred more intimate activities.

I think that's one of the things that attracted me to my first bout at escorting.

I've always been reasonably keen on men, but it's very much a passing phase with me.

Bit like eating a Chinese takeaway!

Never full for too long and then you want another one till you get bored with them.

I can take it or leave it as my mood changes.

Anyway I thought why not get paid for something I enjoyed.

Mandy goes on the game!

<u>Escorting</u>
Okay I know this has nothing to do with my second visit, but it gives you a bit more of a flavour to my lifestyle prior to meeting Misty.

Not all TVs are like this by the way - just working gurlz like me!

I initially put an advert on one of the TV sites with an escort section, and all the business came from there.

It was quite a reasonable fee for the year, as it only cost 25 pounds, and you could alter the text and pictures as many times as you liked.

Now, Lincolnshire is not a thriving metropolis, and there's not exactly a lot of money round here, as the main employment seems to be connected to agriculture.

But that seemed to work in my favour, as there aren't a lot of TV escorts either.

There wasn't much competition in terms of professional Lincolnshire gurlz, and I didn't look too bad compared to those who did advertise.

I thought I stood a fair chance, so I put the advert in and drew a few punters.

Well, to be honest it was money for old rope, especially if they were newcomers.

They booked an hour for 100 pounds but were only with me for ten minutes.

Easy come, easy go, as they say!

Okay, so it took me about twenty minutes to get ready, when I had it down to a fine art, but it seemed a reasonable way to earn a few bob.

I know it's always risky working alone, but I built up a regular client base and never really had any trouble, apart from one client who was a little bit weird.

I spoke to him on the phone, and he seemed like he was a real gentleman and said he was going to call in on his way up to Scotland. Think he was going on holiday to see his son and daughter-in-law.

When he arrived he was nothing like his pictures on Chix. His picture must have been about twenty years out of date. Like I said there's a lot of misleading pictures on Chix, but we got on okay. I showed him into the lounge, and we had a reasonable conversation.

He seemed quite articulate, and we did all the usual flimflam and soon headed for the bedroom.

In the bedroom things were not as they normally are with most punters, who come and go in quick succession, if you follow my drift.

This one had a particular kinky fantasy. I could probably have said no, but I already had his 100 pounds in my pocket so I listened to his request.

His fantasy was to make me cry - like a real girl!

Nothing vicious, but he applied some pressure in certain vulnerable places until he got the desired result.

Well, it didn't last that long, and I guess in terms of what you hear some gurlz go through it was fairly minor in comparison. Actually I quite enjoyed it if I'm truthful. Did make me feel a little more gurly.

I just know I was bloody sore for a while afterwards though.

New balls, please!

At that time I was working from home, but it was getting complicated with my son, as I had to make sure he was out. I looked elsewhere for suitable accommodation and found some which I tried for a while.

I knew a transsexual in Lincoln and used to use her house occasionally. It was a four-storey house with a cellar underneath that she'd turned into a fully equipped dungeon.

The other floors were bedrooms, and one room was a schoolroom where she used to take lessons for naughty boys.

I used to ring her when I had a prospective client and make arrangements to pop over and gave her a share of the profits afterwards.

It was fine for a while, but I gave up in the end as she turned out to be unreliable.

I remember one Sunday I'd arranged to meet one of my clients there who was paying me the usual 100 pounds for the visit.

I made all the arrangements for me to go over and get changed and told the client what time to arrive.

When I got there on the Sunday morning the house was all locked up and she was nowhere to be seen. I tried her on her mobile, but that went straight through to an answer phone.

Found out later that she'd gone over to Lancashire to meet another transsexual and got wasted on the Saturday night.

I ended up having to ring the client to cancel the appointment and never saw him again, so I wasn't too pleased in light of all the running around I'd done for nothing.

Never went back there again.

Following that I made enquiries elsewhere and eventually found myself at a brothel on the outskirts of Boston. It was an old church that had been converted inside and was a real swanky pad.

The owner was a lovely down-to-earth girl who was dressed in a tracksuit and just answered the phone all day. She was obviously doing okay as she had a BMW sports car parked in the drive.

I had a long chat with her, and she said I could rent a room for a fee, but she'd have to give first priority to her girls.

That was okay, but the rent was quite expensive, and on the times I tried to arrange a few appointments she was fully booked. I didn't like having to ring clients back and forth to arrange and rearrange things.

In the end I decided the only option was to work from home again. At least that gave me more control. I'd just have to be very careful as far as my son was concerned.

One thing I didn't want was him coming home to see me dressed with a client in the house.

He knew about Mandy, as I left my computer open one day on a TV website, but he'd never seen me dressed and certainly didn't know about the escorting side of things.

I didn't really want him to get too much of an idea of how Daddy was making a living at that time.

Mandy in Tart Mode

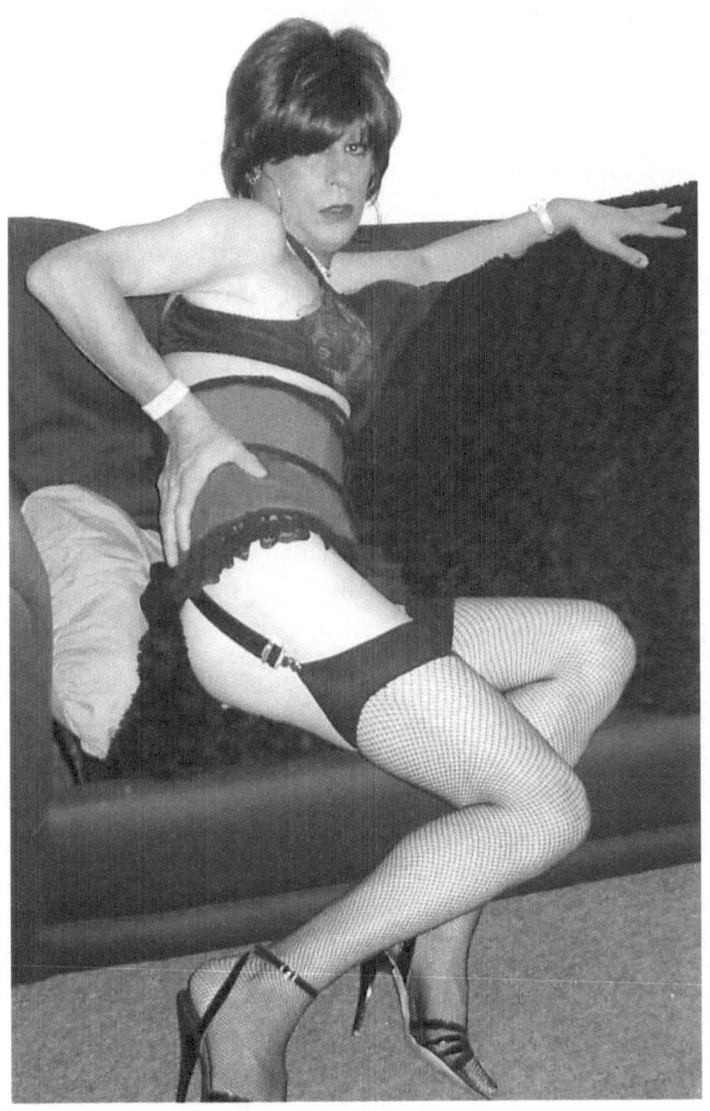

Going back to my second visit to Misty's, it took me about the same time to get ready as it had last Saturday, so it must have been knocking on for about seven before I came downstairs again.

We sat and chatted for a while and drank a few glasses of wine, and Misty rolled a few joints to take with her.

All the same touchy-feely stuff was there, just like it had been last weekend.

Seemed like the magic was still there.

Didn't feel like I had been away and time with Misty was so easygoing that it just drifted by as if nothing else in the world mattered.

As I was staying two nights, Misty wanted us to go to the Philbeach on Saturday.

Seemed like it was going to be a full weekend.

Before we knew it was nearly nine, so Misty suggested we better go if we were going to arrive at a reasonable time.

Although it was April it was still cold in the evenings, and Misty asked me what I was going to wear over my dress.

Bedroom gurlz don't have coats!

I was just going to wear my dress.

Misty suggested I borrow her foxy fur coat, which was hanging in the hall.

I loved it and still have it to this day.

I had my 5-inch heels on and thought I better be honest and say there was no way I could walk far in them.

They were real killers!

They'd really only been worn inside and normally in a bedroom.

Tart!

So she said she would go and bring the car round to the back of her house. I always remember thinking how nice that was of her.

Always considerate.

Getting the car was always a bit of a ritual, as she didn't want to draw too much attention to herself.

I knew she had her own business and kept herself to herself, but it was a close-knit community, and she had a lot of friendly neighbours. Very much of an east-end type community spirit round there.

The back of her house had a small yard with a barbeque and table and chairs. We'd often sit out there (*en drab*) having a drink and chat to the neighbours as they passed by.

One neighbour, who lived about three doors up, used to often bring leftover food round for Eddy and make a fuss of him.

She always struck me as a gentle lady, in contrast to her two sons, who are both dead now.

Ronnie and Reginald!

Anyway, Misty changed her shoes back into her flat loafers and put her other shoes in a carrier bag. Must admit she looked a bit funny being all tarted up with flat shoes on. When the coast was clear she sneaked out to get the car.

Tranny goes walkabout!

I had strict instructions to keep an eye on Eddy, as he used to play this little game when he knew she was going out. As soon as he saw the back door open he'd make a beeline for it and go and hide somewhere outside.

Of course if he did that we couldn't leave till he came back. We couldn't exactly go chasing after him dressed the way we were.

I wonder if he knew?

I offered to go with her, but being the gurl she was she said no, as she didn't want me to walk all that way.

She brought the car round so I could climb straight into the passenger seat, which was something I'll always remember.

I was sitting there beside her with Chris Rea on the stereo. One hand was somewhere it shouldn't be, and I snuggled up beside her, while we sped up the M1 towards Milton Keynes.

She had a few jays on the way. Misty said she knew where it was, but it had been so long since she had been there that we got lost and it took us about an hour and a half to get there.

The car park was full, so we ended up parking across the road in the Campanile car park and did the dreaded steep verge.

Had to hold onto some trees and each other and got both our heels covered in mud, but we found the firm ground eventually and clicked our heels across the road to PP.

The club was absolutely heaving, and we checked in and went upstairs to the bar to get some drinks. I kept Misty's fur coat on as it felt divine.

Fur coat and knickers - LOL!

We met a few gurlz there who we both knew. There was Jackie, UK Mandy, and Jackie Fender.

Misty and I quite liked Jackie Fender, and she suggested we play with her later, but we never found her again in all the crowds.

Most of the night we just sat together and chatted. We said hello to people as they passed by, but to all intents and purposes no one else seemed to matter to us that night.

I was just so glad to be there on Misty's arm.

Felt like I was showing her off, but then she'd said the same thing about taking me there.

I remember there were lots of gurlz there of all ages and sizes, and I knew most of them would probably be looking for a fumble somewhere, but still be going home alone.

Being a TV can be a very lonely occupation!

I felt I was the luckiest gurl in the world when we left.

Misty and me on our first BNO

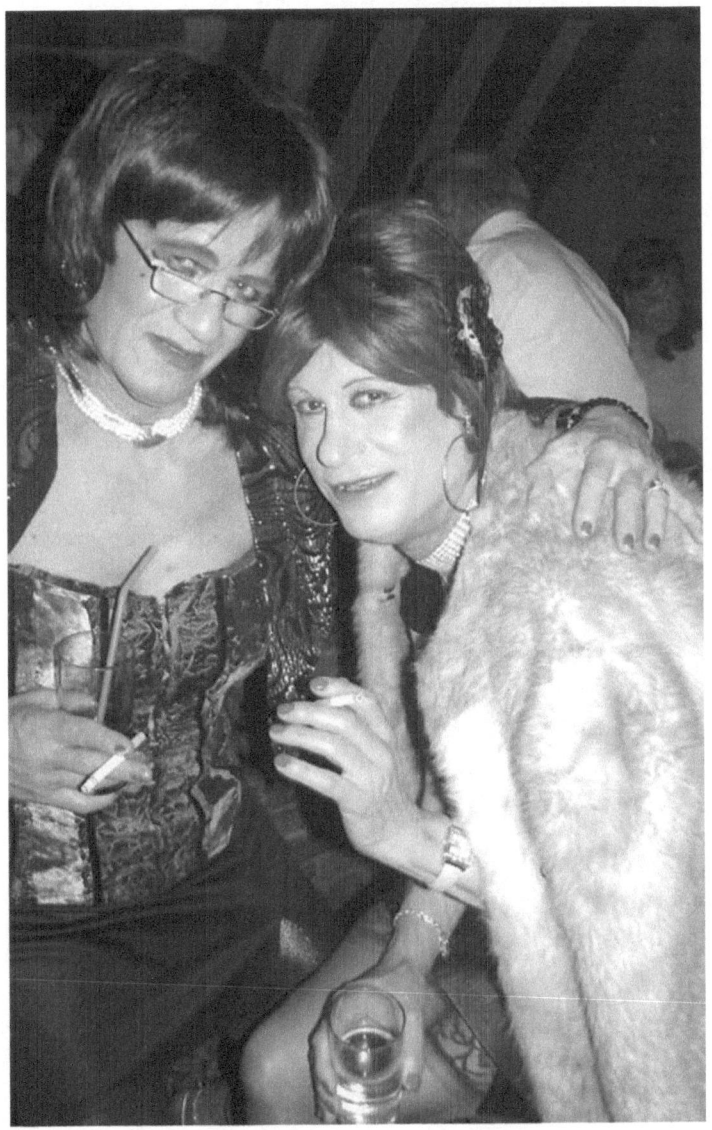

We didn't leave till closing. Misty had a joint and we got lost, but I didn't care. I just sat there purring beside her.

Back at Misty's we sat up till the early morning listening to some music and having a few more drinks and cuddling each other.

It must have been about seven before we snuggled up in Misty's bed again and held on to each other till we dropped off.

The feeling of her lying close to me again was just as it had been on that first night. Well, the honest word was bliss. No other word for it!

I guess the only downside was that we both stayed dressed for the night.

Lingerie and wigs.

Don't think either of us dared spoil the illusion by taking them off at that stage. I guess for many TVs that's all they'll ever know, but it was enough for now.

We didn't get up early the next day and spent most of the day just lazing about until it was time to get fully dressed to go out in the evening. As I said previously Misty wanted to take me to the Philbeach.

Being partially dressed all day felt a bit stilted, but I was so besotted that I really didn't care.

All I wanted was to spend as much time with Misty as was possible.

Late in the afternoon I had a bath, got shaved, and did my makeup.

I had to put my halter neck on again with my 5-inch heels. Misty lent me her coat again, and when we were both ready she went to get the car, which she brought to the back door.

Off to the Phily again!

Diversion at the Philbeach

I had stayed at the Philbeach about a year ago on one contract, so it was nice to be going there again. It brought back some fond memories.

Needless to say the Phily was a tranny hotel.

Going back I'd been doing a contract in London, and during the first week I commuted down there each day from Grantham, which was killing me. I used to get up at four thirty in the morning and then not get home again until eight in the evening.

I needed somewhere to stay and had heard about the Philbeach, so I booked in there.

I remember packing my suitcase before I left. It was so full with women's stuff that I could only just squeeze a couple of clean shirts and socks on top.

I spent that Monday in the office with my suitcase right beside me, desperately hoping it didn't get nicked by someone.

Would have been a little embarrassing to say the least!

When four thirty came I got the tube over to Earls Court and set off to find the hotel.

Being somewhat stupid, I had the map the wrong way up and walked the wrong way out of the tube station, wondering why I couldn't find the hotel.

Doh!

It was a good half hour before I eventually found my way back to the hotel.

I recognised it from the picture on the web with its little triangular red awning over the steps leading into the front.

When I got to the hotel I checked into one of the two rooms behind reception, which were both double rooms with a loo and a shower each.

Anyone who has stayed there knows that most of rooms are single with small washbasins but no baths or toilettes.

Well, a double cost a bit more, but I thought if I was staying for a week I wanted somewhere to wash. I hated the idea of sharing a loo.

Not very gurly!

Of course Monday night at the Philbeach was a gurlz night.

They put on a small buffet in the bar, and the place got packed with gurlz and admirers.

Even back then my favourite dress was my black and white halter neck and the same old strappy black sandals, except that in those days I had a different wig.

It was what Misty called my "flossie" look. Well, I got changed and filled my handbag and then tottered off to the restaurant, which was just round the corner from my room.

It was called the Thai Princess and was run by Jade, who dressed *en femme* and served all the guests.

I felt very nervous sitting there for the first time by myself, but the staff were lovely and very friendly, and a few glasses of wine soon relaxed me.

Must have been about nine when I finished, so I paid the bill and found my way down to the bar, where all the TVs and admirers were gathered.

It was absolutely packed, so I made my way across to the bar and ordered a drink from Jimmy, who was the Scottish barman and something of a local character.

There were a lot of gurlz there who must have been regulars as they knew each other, so I felt a bit like a fish out of water not knowing anyone. Felt like a real wallflower.

Anyway, I clung to the bar with a drink in one hand and a cigarette in the other. Hoping to look nonchalant!

You can usually tell when it's someone's first time!

One pretty gurl in a party dress kept brushing past and touching me gently on several occasions, making it fairly obvious that she fancied me.

Jane!

Anyway, we eventually got talking and she asked me to go and sit with her.

I felt accepted at last.

Trouble was she was there with her boyfriend so had to behave that night, but we became firm friends and I met her on a later date.

Well, nothing happened on that first night, and I went to bed alone, but I can honestly say that after that I had company every night.

Nudge nudge - wink wink - say no more!

Most of the gurlz I met were very nice, and there was even one who met me one night as an admirer and then the next night as a gurl.

Best of both worlds.

When I say most were nice, there were also some really weird ones. I met a couple of gurlz who were staying there who seemed to be way off balance.

They had some really weird fantasies!

Towards the end of my second week I met Karen, who was a real hoot. She was a broad Geordie foreman who was working on the tubes.

I met her in the bar, where she was already well smashed, but we got on well. I took her back to my room, where she soon threw up.

Drink was another big thing in the TV world. She blamed it on something Jimmy had given her to drink:

Like a bottle of vodka!

We kept in contact for ages, and last time I heard from her she had just been let out by the police. She was living with some girl who was a bit of druggie and the girl had thrown herself out of her bathroom window (second storey flat).

Karen got blamed and got locked up by the police, but fortunately the girl recovered and told them the truth. That was typical of the sort of scrapes she used to get into!

After my contract ended I went back to Lincolnshire but had arranged to come down again in a few weeks.

The plan was to meet an admirer at the Philbeach and then spend the following night at the Beaver with Jane.

The Beaver is a hotel just a few doors down from the Philbeach.

Tranny friendly.

The admirer was a Scottish guy who was a freelance journalist and used to fly down to London quite often.

Something to do with Football.

He said he'd get down in the late afternoon, but he also rang the hotel to arrange to let me have access to the room earlier so I could change.

He booked a nice double room at the Philbeach with a bathroom and toilette and a big brass bed. I got there about two o'clock and got changed into my bedroom gear.

Black piegnoire - très chique.

He arrived at about six o'clock, and we did what you normally do. Straight off the plane from Scotland.

A wash might have been nice - LOL!

Then I got dressed for dinner, and we wandered down to the restaurant.

Think I actually wore a different dress on this occasion. It was a brown dress which I bought in Boston. A young female assistant said the colour would suit me.

Guess it's a woman's intuition!

Dinner in the Thai restaurant is always good, and the admirer paid for everything as he had said he would.

Kept woman!

Think that was part of the turn-on for him. He didn't seem too interested in the other stuff. Just wanted to be seen out and about with me and make sure everyone knew he was footing the bill.

The staff fussed round him, and I got the impression he was something of a celebrity. Of course it didn't mean a thing to me.

Do I look like football fan?

After dinner we went down to the bar and got started on the whiskies. Being Scottish, he had some gifts for Jimmy, which included haggis. The bar was quiet that night, so Jimmy joined us and we all got rat-arsed together.

There was a lot of nostalgic talk about Scotland, and then we moved on to Jimmy's hobby.

Jimmy (or James) must have been in his mid-fifties and had been at the Phily since the year dot. He was a tall thin guy who often wore full Scottish regalia.

Gay Gordon - well, Gay Jimmy!

Jimmy's main hobby was taking pictures of tombstones. I say "main" because it involved a little bit more than that!

Let's just say Jimmy used to take his young lovers home, and the rumour is that they were often involved in some of the more graphic night time pictures taken with a self timer.

Anyway, when the bar closed we went back up to bed and what I thought would be some more cavorting.

Well, he'd want his money's worth!

The earlier evening playtime had been relatively light, so I assumed more was to follow. After a short cuddle he just turned over and went to sleep.

I was quite grateful, as I wasn't really in the mood for further hanky-panky.

Didn't like his beard too much - plays havoc with the makeup!

In the morning he had to go out to work, so he left me to my own devices. I stayed as long as I could until they kicked me out, and then wandered down to the Beaver.

It was TV friendly as long as you weren't too obvious about it, and the rooms were a lot better. They all had showers.

Enter Jane!

Jane arrived about four o'clock, and it was the first time I had seen her undressed. It was not normally something she liked doing.

I know when she met her admirer she always arrived and left dressed and used to sort herself out in the car. She used to use lay-bys and got some funny looks from passing reps who were probably wishing it was them getting changed.

Think she had something of a complicated life, as she had a wife, a girlfriend, and an admirer.

FFS!

I knew her wife knew nothing about her lifestyle, and she used to keep everything stored in locked containers in the garage, where she restored old cars.

She also used to race sidecars as well, which seemed a bit of a departure from this lifestyle.

I remember she said she was in the defence industry and often had to go away and couldn't even tell her wife where she was going.

Top secret and all that!

That always seemed like a cracking good excuse for this type of activity.

Didn't even have to lie!

We got dressed together and then set off for dinner at the Philbeach.

As I said, it wasn't a long walk, but when you've got your 5-inch heels on it was a bit of killer. Had a lovely dinner and a bottle of wine before going down to see Jimmy and whoever else was around.

That's when we met the lovely Myra!

Oh, boy! Was she a nut - but a lot of transsexuals are!

We were in two minds about her, but it was late and getting on for closing time, and in the end she came back with us to the Beaver. Not sure if we invited her or if she invited herself.

Well, we got back and she had real delusions about herself. She wasn't much to look at and had big staring scary eyes.

Said she was a porn star and kept asking us to tell her how beautiful she was. Think she was a bit obsessed with her bust. Bottom half hadn't been done at that stage. Couldn't get her out of there fast enough.

Porn star - LMAO! (laughing my arse off) - she's only a hooker now!

Jane has been a firm friend ever since, and we've kept in contact on a regular basis.

She even came up to party in Lincoln.

I talked to Jane a lot on Yahoo!, and I remember she told me how her admirer had dumped her. She'd been seeing him for about three years and done most of London with him.

I know she was devastated - in floods of tears!

I know that seems strange, as she also had a wife and a girlfriend, but as I said before:

It's never black and white in our world!

Anyway, to get back to the main story, that Friday.

It took us about half an hour to get there, and Misty dropped me off outside the door and went to park the car.

I stayed in the entrance till Misty came, and then we both went down to the bar for a couple of drinks before dinner.

The irrespirable James was there, and he remembered me from my previous visits, even though I'd changed my wig.

We had a great evening and met a few people we both knew. I know it sounds corny, but at dinner we really only had eyes for each other. We even held hands across the table.

LOL - very romantic!

We left when it was closing time and walked back to the car. I snuggled into my seat and listened to Chris Rea on the way back.

It was *On the Beach*, which has some songs that have a special meaning to me now.

With the combination of the drink, the music, and Misty beside me, I couldn't have asked for more.

The one thing I haven't mentioned until now is sex!

When I first met her I had no idea how much she played about, but I assumed she'd been round the block a few more times than me.

In truth she hadn't really played around that much and was much more of a flirt who enjoyed the chase rather than actually getting there.

Anyway, I was pretty much in love with her by this stage, despite it only being my second visit.

None of her past experiences mattered to me.

If you really want to know what happened between us, all I can say is she never screwed me in the way most other gurlz and admirers do.

We made love!

We just seemed to connect in a way I'd never thought possible with anyone. We got very intimate that night.

It must have been about six in the morning before we went to bed. Misty was curled up behind me holding me tight as I drifted off without a care in the world.

On Sunday morning I got up early again, got changed, and said goodbye fairly quickly. It wasn't because I wanted to go, as I would have stayed all week if I had the option.

I guess it was because this was only my second visit, and something told me inside that Misty wanted some space.

I was right and I found out later that on most Sunday mornings Misty used to feel like that.

She used to switch off.

She told me it was because she knew I'd be gone soon and she'd feel sad and empty.

Her way of shutting it all out till next time!

<u>Monday 16 to Friday 20 April</u>
I talked to Misty most evenings that next week on Yahoo!.
It wasn't every day, and to be honest, when I was online
in the evening and she didn't come on I used to worry
like anything.

I always had visions of her in her cottage in London still
playing the field. Anyway, in the end I arranged to go
and see Misty on Saturday, and she said we'd go to the
Philbeach for dinner.

<u>Friday 20 and Saturday 21 April</u>
In the end I couldn't make the Saturday, and I think
Misty may have had some things she needed to sort out
with the new business.

Anyway, before we met she had previously arranged to go
and see Carole and Tanya in High Wycombe for a little
party. When we realised we couldn't meet she said she'd
be there in the evening.

With everything we'd shared so far I was a bit gutted, but
I didn't let her know that.

Despite her email from the first week, I felt like I was just
another gurl in a long stream.

Maybe I shouldn't take it all so seriously after all.

Stupid tart!

I remember what I said at the beginning. Gurlz don't really fall in love, and maybe I was just fooling myself about it all.

I'd only met her twice, and as much as I wanted to be her gurl, I always knew she'd play around a bit.

She made it fairly clear at our first meeting that she was something of a predator and that it went with the territory.

Leopards never change their spots!

Maybe it was just wishful thinking on my behalf. Anyway, we spoke on Saturday lunchtime on the phone.

Misty told me she missed me, and I could tell she meant it, but she was still off to meet Carole in High Wycombe in the evening.

Well, I got a bit jealous and spoke to Carole on Yahoo! and said I might see her on the Sunday, which I told Misty.

I didn't really want to, but I thought it sounded sort of cavalier and said nothing about how much I cared for Misty.

Lovesick puppy!

I was sitting at home on Saturday night thinking about things when Misty rang me from High Wycombe, which she had no need to do.

I think that said a lot - well, it warmed my heart.

I asked her to pass a message on to Carole that I couldn't go on the Sunday, but then I never really intended to.

I know it sounds silly, but I guess that despite everything that was happening, I was already beginning to think of myself as a one-person gurl. Silly sod!

<u>Sunday 22 April</u>
I spoke to Misty, who said the party was okay but Carole got pissed quite early.

She was apparently miffed that Misty and Tanya started playing together without her, and I think that put her nose out of joint.

Misty had mentioned that Tanya might be there and said she nearly knocked her out.

Apparently Tanya had brought some duty free cigarettes for Misty, and she paid her for them but was a pound short.

Misty found a pound in her bag and jokingly lobbed it at Tanya.

Smacked her right between the eyes!

All my misgivings just seemed to disappear when I talked to her. She had a knack of doing that.

Didn't seem to matter what or who had happened.

She was very infectious in that way.

She said she wanted to meet next weekend, and I got quite excited about that. It would be my third time of meeting her, and it was almost becoming a regular event.

I still wasn't working and was seriously thinking about going back to escorting again just to earn a few extra pennies.

I wasn't sure what Misty might think about it, so I decided I'd drop it into the conversation the next weekend and see what her reaction was.

Things were getting a little urgent, so during the week I started putting out some feelers and ended up going to see Cindy in Skegness with a view to setting up an escorting business.

Cindy was okay but not really my cup of tea. Anyway, I went over to meet her and ended up in bed just to show that I was willing and let her see the goods. Got well screwed I guess. But business is business!

Someone has to do it - LOL!

I could have worked from home as I had before, but it made a lot of sense to work with someone else as added protection.

You never know who's going to walk through the door. In addition I had my son living with me, so it wouldn't really be fair on him.

<u>Saturday 28 April</u>
I arranged to go and see Misty on the Saturday and drove down as excited as anything.

We went to the Philbeach that night, as we'd previously arranged. Of course when we went there Misty usually paid for everything. The meal and all the drinks.

She really looked after me.

It was a quiet night with not many gurlz about. We had a drink in the bar first, said hello to a few people, chatted to James, and then went to the restaurant at about nine.

We sat in a table in the corner and talked like lovers, holding hands across the table again.

Pretty oblivious to anything else.

Soppy or what!

There was an old gay guy sitting behind us. He was dressed in a suit and looked quite smart. Think he was an economics lecturer in one of the London colleges.

I say gay guy as opposed to admirer as he didn't have too much time for gurlz. He had a very dry and sarcastic sense of humour and he'd had a few verbal fisticuffs with Misty in the past (humorous).

Anyway, he said hello and they had a bit of banter and then he asked how long we'd known each other. Misty said only a few weeks, and he was taken aback.

Said he was surprised as we looked so comfortable together. He said he thought we must have known each other for ages. Felt very good to hear that.

Wasn't just me wishing it, then!

Anyway, at some stage I thought I better mention the escorting, so I dropped it into the conversation. Misty was very cool about it.

Well, she appeared to be.

She mentioned she had a friend from whom she'd borrowed her name. She was an Anglo-Burmese gurl who was an escort. Misty had helped out on a few occasions and had made up numbers when the clients wanted a threesome.

Her response made me feel a lot better, but in all honesty all I really wanted to know was that she cared for me a little and I wouldn't have minded if she had said no.

I really didn't like the thought of doing all that grubby work again.

It just seemed all so incongruous in comparison to the gurl I was smitten with.

After dinner we went to the bar, and James the barman said something similar to the old gay guy's remark. We didn't leave till the bar closed, and we drove back to Misty's and snuggled up on the sofa.

It was always lovely to go out and show off but even better to get home.

It must have been about five in the morning before we crashed out. Felt so safe and content in that big bed and it seemed my refuge from the world. Nothing could harm me there.

Eddy was starting to accept me by now and was happy to get up on my lap, which was an honour.

He usually runs a mile with strangers.

By now all three of us that went to bed. Eddy used to sleep on the pillows in between our heads.

No pussy jokes - LOL!

Got home on Sunday, and as I didn't have much money at the time I threw myself into escorting and organizing adverts.

I had an old escort site on BirchPlace from my times before, so I reactivated that and got a bit of business. Also went over to see Cindy, as we had a few appointments there.

They were really yucky, but they earned a few pennies. I had a phone call from this client in Birmingham. I said it was too far to travel, as it was about 100 miles. He just kept ringing and ringing, so I agreed in the end.

Misty knew about it and phoned me while I was driving there. She wished me good luck and told me to be careful.

I didn't drive dressed, which the client knew, so he left the door ajar. I went straight into the bathroom to get changed so he didn't see the drab me.

As it was only a moderate class hotel, the bathroom was minute. With me and my case I could hardly turn round. I managed it in the end and went out to see the client, who was only a really young guy.

I just couldn't figure out why he wanted to pay for it.

Guess it's a turn-on to some guys!

Think they get some weird kick out of thinking they own your Ass for a while. Anyway, it only lasted two hours.

I made 100 pounds from that and with other appointments had a bit of cash.

Cindy had copied some of my piccies and put them on Chix under her profile. I was livid about it, especially as she captioned one of the piccies:

"My girlfriend - FFS!"

I told her to take them off, and she said she would. I just hoped Misty wouldn't spot them in the meantime.

Well, she did and went ballistic about it!

I had to ring Cindy and tell her again in no uncertain terms. Fortunately it didn't spoil things between me and Misty, but you can imagine what I was thinking at the time.

Normal relationships can be fragile in the early days, but TV relationships are even worse. Because it's all conducted in secrecy and there's so much sex drive it's sometimes so hard to know how others will react to any small change. Can be like walking in a minefield at times.

I think she knew it was only business and Cindy had got hold of the wrong end of the stick.

<u>Saturday 5 May</u>

It was a bank holiday weekend, and last week Misty had told me she was planning on having a party and wanted me to come down and co-host it with her. I arranged to go down on the Saturday and got there at about twelve.

There were going to be about eight of us all together: me, Misty, Susan, Jackie, Sabrina, Simone, Debbs, and Tina.

I'd been to a couple of parties before but felt a little bit nervous about this one.

I wasn't sure what Misty expected of me, and in truth all I really wanted was to be with her, so I was treading on eggshells a bit.

As far as I knew Misty was still a gurl about town, and a bit promiscuous, so I thought the best way to impress her was to take a chance and throw myself into it.

Not that I needed much encouragement!

Once a trollop always a trollop!

I'd see what happened afterwards and just hope I got it right!

The first guests arrived at about seven.

It was Susan and Jackie.

Susan went upstairs to dress, and Jackie, who was already dressed, sat downstairs with me and Misty.

Then Sabrina turned up *en* drab and was about to get changed downstairs in front of us all. That was the first time I'd been in the same room when Misty lost her cool.

She told Sabrina it was out of order and that she'd have to change upstairs.

She got quite cross, which is not surprising, as it would have been really naff for Sabrina to change in front of everyone else.

Not really the done thing in a room full of trannies.

It doesn't really work!

Sabrina went upstairs to dress, and in the meantime Susan came down dressed.

Misty made sure the drink was flowing, and I guess with one thing and another I started the party.

I sat beside Jackie on the sofa, and one thing led to another, as they do.

I think you can guess the rest!

At this point Simone turned up (*en femme*), and she told Misty she was quite impressed to arrive at a party where everything (in other words, me and Jackie) was in full swing.

Misty always regarded Simone as a "Premiere league" gurl who she quite fancied, so she took that as a great compliment.

Premiere league means just what it says. Someone out of the top drawer in terms of looks and poise.

Soon all the guests turned up. The last to arrive were Debbs and Tina. Sabrina was about to start on Simone, and I remember watching as Misty suddenly pulled her to one side and said "I'm pulling rank."

I remember I looked over and had a real pang of jealousy run through me as Misty and Simone got acquainted.

I tried to concentrate on what (or who) I was doing, but it tied my heart in knots and I had a little pit in my stomach.

C'est la vie!

Not going into graphic detail, but everyone got pissed or stoned, and I was given a nickname that stuck.

Moaning Manders - not a quiet gurl!

Not sure what time it was, but eventually some people left, and in the early morning the rest of us crashed out.

Debbs and Sabrina slept downstairs, while Misty and I slept in the bed upstairs. Susan was already there, as she had zonked out earlier.

I left at about lunchtime on Sunday morning and have to admit I didn't feel that great. Massive hangover and felt like death warmed up.

But more than that, I still wanted to be Misty's gurl and didn't feel so special anymore.

Went home feeling really dejected.

I guess everything works two ways, because a while later Misty told me she had pangs of jealousy when she saw me with the other gurlz.

Wish she'd told me at the time.

Funny, but in our little world you need to do certain things to discover what's really there behind all the glitter.

I guess we did feel the same way about each other.

The rest was just sex with strangers!

Next week, however, Misty mentioned she'd had a mail from a real top notch Premiere league gurl called Georgia. I know Misty wanted to see seen out with her, if only for the kudos!

She was a high-flying accountant for a multinational company and worked abroad but was coming back to England for a couple of weeks.

She'd been in touch, and they'd arranged to meet up at the Phily. I didn't tell Misty, but as far as I was concerned Georgia was no Premiere league gurl.

I knew a little bit about her history and some people she'd associated with, and it was nothing to write home about.

I have to admit I was jealous of Georgia and of any other gurlz who Misty might meet.

Jealousy isn't in my nature, but I'd met someone special who I really cared for a lot, and it seemed reciprocated.

A rare thing in the tranny world!

In truth it broke my heart, but then I knew it went with the territory.

As it turned out, she never actually met Georgia, as she never got over here.

<u>Friday 11 May</u>
I arranged to go down on Friday, as Misty wanted us to go to PP again for the Big Night Out. I got there and changed in the early evening, and Misty did the usual thing of bringing the car round to the back door for me. We didn't get there till about ten thirty, and as usual it was packed.

As usual the car park was full, so we parked across the road in the Campanile car park and had to put the car on a pavement, as that was full as well.

We spent most of the evening upstairs just sitting and chatting to each other. I remember we met Vamps (an RG), and she arranged to give me a wig stand which she had brought with her.

There were quite a few gurlz we knew. We even bumped into Sabrina, who was there with Mandy from London.

Sabrina said she'd pop round on Saturday with the party pictures. She'd got them from all the other gurlz and had about seventy of them on disk.

Cindy had said she might turn up, and eventually she came with Amy and Joanne.

They didn't turn up till one, as they had gotten lost on the way. We just were about to go.

Cindy looked as rough as anything and sat in a corner smoking. Amy chatted to Misty, and they exchanged phone numbers and Yahoo! addresses and tentatively arranged to meet.

I felt the usual pangs of jealousy, as I always did, but nothing would ever come of them.

Simon was there and was well-known as the resident photographer. He took some pictures of everyone, which were later posted on the Big Night Out website.

Think it's what most gurlz went for. TVs are by definition a vain lot!

"My and my best friend at BNO - FFS!"

In the end we didn't leave till about two thirty, and Misty drove us back to London. She was a bit stoned, and we got lost again but eventually found the M1.

The road was almost empty, and we stayed in the middle lane, overtaking the odd lorry and listening to some driving music.

I sat there with my legs on the dashboard and was a bit naughty as I knew the lorry drivers could see them.

They could see right into the car, and I did wonder if they actually knew what they were looking at.

Misty said they knew - a lot of horns were tooted that night - LOL!

You might be surprised at how many TVs and admirers drive big rigs.

We got back at about four in the morning and spent a couple of hours drinking and getting intimate till about six.

It was just like the first time.

It was the same magic and a very dreamy and romantic night. Upstairs I fell asleep with Misty's arms around my waist.

Believe it or not, we still got up relatively early on Saturday and were full of energy.

Sabrina turned up in the late morning *en* drab. She looked the worse for wear but had brought the party pictures with her.

We sat and chatted for a while, and then Misty decided she wanted to pop to the shops later so went back upstairs to change into drab.

That was a big thing, as I had never seen Misty *en* drab.

In fact no one had before - was a closely guarded secret.

I guess it was just one of those times when she just decided to take the bull by the horns and see what my reaction was.

Tranny becomes a bloke!

She wasn't away long, and I waited with bated breath as I heard her come down the stairs. It was May but quite warm outside, so she appeared in a sweatshirt and shorts and some leather loafers.

Well, it had to be, if there was ever going to be any kind of relationship between us, other than purely for dressing and sex.

There was no other option!

Well, if you want my honest reaction it took me all of about one second to accept it.

You never know what to expect, but actually I thought she looked quite good as a guy.

She was what you call a mature gurl (well sixty three), so she was a bit thin on top but looked distinguished.

Just seemed like it was the right thing to do, and I have to admit I'd been waiting for it.

Broke one barrier!

I guess it made me feel a lot more relaxed now that she seemed to think I could accept her the way she was.

Misty asked Sabrina if she'd like to come with us to the Philbeach that night, but she was so hung over that she said no and disappeared.

We went off to Tesco just to get some cat food and coffee. I know it doesn't sound like much, but it meant there was a chance we could develop as real people.

We went to the Philly again that night. It was a wonderful night, and we seemed a lot closer, which I guess was something to do with me having seen and accepted her undressed.

Misty had previously arranged for Tanya to come over the following weekend and that was still on.

Tanya lived in Ibiza, where she worked in a bar, and it would be the last opportunity she'd get before the holiday season started.

She asked me how I felt about the three of us. I wasn't too sure but just said it was fine. Couldn't say much else!

Well, I was worried!

I had seen some pictures of Tanya, and she looked absolutely stunning. Not bad for an ex-paratrooper!

When the Philly closed we drove back to Misty's and got there at about two. She parked the car in a side street, a couple of minutes away from her house.

Misty gets sussed!

Now normally when we came back the streets were deserted, but on this occasion one of her neighbours was walking back from another house.

She was a middle-aged West Indian woman who normally stopped to chat when Misty was sitting in the yard.

I think she must have been to a party.

I suspect she already knew about Misty, but certainly that night left her in no doubt!

We'd already started walking down the lane that runs up to the back of the house, and she was coming the other way. Other than turn round we didn't have much option but to keep going.

Misty said nothing, but I could tell she was feeling very awkward about it. The lady had a puzzled look as she got closer.

Just as we were about to meet we suddenly turned right into the yard, and Misty made a bolt for the door.

The lady said nothing, but as Misty unlocked the door we could sense that she had stopped dead in her tracks.

You could feel her eyes on stalks by then!

We saw her a few weekends later. As normal she stopped to chat, so I think she and the rest of the neighbours just accepted it.

When we got inside Misty poured some stiff drinks. I guess it all added to the excitement of the night, so we ended up getting intimate.

By now I hated going to bed on Saturdays because I knew what was coming on Sunday morning.

I knew I'd soon fall asleep and then in the morning I would have to go.

On that Sunday morning Misty said, "Well, back to reality."

Over for another week!

I clung onto Misty, thinking about the next weekend, and feeling jealous of Tanya!

Just kept thinking she might take her away from me and it would all be over.

Stupid, I know.

But you think these things when you have someone precious.

<u>Friday 18 May</u>
I went down on Friday as I still wasn't working, and after we'd eaten I had a bath and got dressed. We stayed in together and had a lovely time.

I was still nervous about Saturday, but I didn't dare show it.

On Saturday morning we both went off to Tesco to get some food. Tanya arrived on Saturday afternoon.

She had all the confidence you'd expect from someone who'd spent her life working in a bar abroad in her normal mode.

As a woman - well top half!

But she was nice, and all three of us got on very well. I could tell she wasn't going to take Misty away, but I was still felt the usual pangs.

Well, it's only natural.

Misty and I were both *en* drab. We got changed in the late afternoon, and then we all set off to the Phily.

I knew Misty fancied her (well everyone did), so I just acted as cool as I could and made out like I didn't care that much.

Not very convincing, but I put on a brave face.

We got to the Phily and went to the bar downstairs. We sat on each side of Tanya and had some piccies taken. They were a bit page three!

At about nine we went upstairs and had a meal in the restaurant. Sabrina turned up with Jackie and they joined us.

Misty was in a party mood and suggested they both come back to her place. When the Phily closed Jackie drove her own car, but Sabrina came with us.

That was a very unpleasant journey, as Sabrina sat between myself and Tanya in the back and had a slight personal problem regarding hygiene.

Misty was sitting in the front and smoking, so she was unaware of it.

What a whiff!

When we got back to Misty's we sat and had a few drinks, but it wasn't a party atmosphere, which I knew Misty had hoped for.

It all fell a bit flat, so Jackie left after a while and made some excuse about having to get up early the next day.

That left just the four of us.

Misty and Tanya went upstairs, which left me downstairs with Sabrina. I wasn't in a party mood either and really didn't want to play with Sabrina.

I didn't fancy her that much, and the hygiene problem really turned me off.

Besides which, I wanted to be with Misty, but I knew she was upstairs playing with Tanya.

I felt as if Misty had excluded me, and it felt very lonely being downstairs then.

To be honest I wished I hadn't drunk so much, and right then I wanted to go home and run away from it all.

Guess some of that was the wine talking.

Always makes me melancholy.

Sabrina thought we could get it on downstairs, and I made an effort, but in the end I just couldn't cope with it anymore. I kept hearing noises from upstairs.

Sabrina knew something was going on, and in the end I just burst into tears and spurted everything out.

Told her I was in love!

She understood it a little, but she was a bit too much of a bloke to understand it properly.

Misty had been smoking jays when we came home, and I guess that was part of it all.

Not really sure if she knew what was happening.

Anyway, Sabrina knew nothing was going to happen between us, and after a while Misty came downstairs. She knew something was up.

She told me later it was the look in my eyes.

My puppy dog look!

Misty sat down, had a drink, and talked to us both. She knew she had to do something which she didn't really like to do.

Basically she told me to go upstairs and join Tanya.

She told Sabrina she couldn't stay the night and ordered her a taxi, which took ages to arrive.

I joined Tanya in bed and we played a bit. She had a lovely body and a very nice bust with nipple rings, which were fun.

When Sabrina left Misty came back upstairs, and all three of us spent the night playing together before we fell asleep.

Three in a bed - yummy!

When we got up on Sunday everyone was in drab except Tanya. She had to get the plane back to Ibiza that night, but she wanted to get some British things from a supermarket that she couldn't get over there.

Misty was cooking lunch for us all, so I suggested that I go with Tanya and show her the way to Tesco.

No one knew what to make of Tanya in the supermarket. They couldn't work out whether they were looking at a gurl or a guy.

If anyone stared she looked straight back with an air of confidence, which always disarms people.

As soon as you do that they look away.

I had to keep my hands in my pockets the whole time, as I still had my red nail varnish on. I was worried about what people might say.

Couldn't give a toss now!

We went back to Misty's. She'd cooked roast beef with all the trimmings, which was great when you could get Eddy out of the way. He was a real little thief and would go for anything.

That included your plate!

Misty and I dressed in the late afternoon. We all chilled out until Tanya had to leave to catch the plane.

Tanya said it was always quiet abroad in the winter, and Misty suggested putting us both in a house and setting us up as London escorts.

That didn't seem a bad idea at the time, and I guess it would have made a fair bit of money. But events overtook us, and it never got off the ground.

After Tanya left I stayed the night. Misty told me she'd been quite jealous when she heard me and Tanya upstairs the previous night.

Goes both ways!

We had a good chat about the weekend and laid a few feelings on the table, as it seemed the right time for it.

It took some time for us to get there, but we did, and we had a wonderful time that night.

I drove back on the Monday and went back to escorting, which I felt bad about. All I wanted was to be with Misty and not all the crappy clients.

I really hated going over there and doing what I did to earn some money.

Tart with a heart I guess!

We had an advert coming out at the weekend. Cindy wanted me to be there, but I said I wasn't prepared to do that.

Not going to sacrifice a weekend with Misty just on the off chance that a punter might turn up.

Most of them were no shows, anyway.

Saw a couple of people at Cindy's, but it was pretty disgusting, and I hated it.

They were big fat and sweaty people who had sneaked out without telling the wives where they were going.

I used to dress in my maid's outfit with my long blonde wig.

Misty said it made me look all frumpy.

Hated to think of the things I did there. I used to dress the guys up, and they got quite excited, so one thing led to another.

Ugh!

Cindy just sat there and smoked while I did all the work, which was a bit cheeky.

And I only got half the money!

Money was still tight. Although my son didn't know the details, he knew I was up to no good and didn't like what he probably suspected I was doing.

I thought I'd go back to contracting so got onto an agency and sorted out a short-term contract.

Even had an admirer sitting next to me on that contract!

It was with British Gas up in Leeds, but it would earn some decent money for a short while.

One night as I was driving back from Cindy's and I'd had enough of it all. I'd already made up my mind to stop it, and Misty texted me and said:

"Please tell me you've stopped escorting."

That really touched me.

It was the first time I realised that she didn't really like it!

I went over to see Cindy for the last time. I told her I was stopping escorting as I'd gotten a contract, which started on Tuesday the twenty-ninth of May, after the bank holiday.

Cindy was okay about it and understood it was because of the money.

<u>Friday 25 May</u>

It was another a bank holiday weekend. I drove down on the Friday and didn't have to come back till the Monday, so that meant three nights with Misty.

I'd been doing about 80 miles an hour all the way down the M1 and then slowed down for the short five miles to Misty's when I pulled up in a parking slot.

Couldn't turn the steering and had no brakes.

Guess I had tart's luck that day!

I panicked then because I knew I had to get the car fixed for Tuesday for work.

Also, I didn't want to miss this long weekend with Misty.

We both had a look at the car but decided to leave it for the night and sort it out on Saturday.

In the end I contacted the breakdown people, who agreed I could ring them on Monday and get it towed back then. Meantime I arranged a hire car for Monday while I got it repaired.

It meant I had the whole weekend with Misty.

Whoopee!

From the Friday night until I left on Monday we spent the whole weekend by ourselves.

Once I got the arrangements for the car sorted on Saturday morning we went into town and Misty took us to a little Italian restaurant.

It was one of her regular watering holes, and she was greeted by the owner like a long lost-friend.

She often went there by herself or with cricketing buddies, so taking me there was a big thing for both of us.

She wanted to see how I behaved in public and how compatible we might be in the outside world. It felt like a big test, but I understood why she needed to do it.

Unfortunately I forgot myself and still thought we were out somewhere like the Philbeach. I suddenly found one of my hands resting on hers on the table! Even she hadn't noticed.

Whoops - camp tart!

Good job no one else saw it. I quickly drew my hand back and reverted to male mode.

The rest of the time we spent in Misty's cottage. It was so relaxed, and time just seemed to drift by in a lovely dream.

Misty said she'd never spent three days in her house with one gurl. I think that was another little test to see how we got on.

Neither of us got bored!

On the Sunday morning Misty did a barbecue on the terrace. We spent the afternoon sitting in the backyard drinking. Eddy slept under a bush.

A few neighbours passed by and stopped to chat at the fence. We just chilled out until it was time to get dressed for the evening.

We just spent it together as we had the previous nights. Drinking and talking and cuddling and generally getting very intimate.

Most of all, what I really liked was sleeping beside her. As it was a long weekend I had three nights with her. Well, her and Eddy.

We always got dressed in the evening, but when bedtime came we both took our wigs off.

Guess that broke another barrier in the bedroom!

<u>Friday 1 June</u>
I started my contract in Leeds that week and was working long hours. I didn't get home till about half seven. I still spoke to Misty most evenings. On the Tuesday I arranged to go down on the Friday straight from work.

We spoke again (on Yahoo!) on Wednesday night. Misty said she was eating and suddenly went very quiet.

There were some expletives at the other end!

Misty snapped a tooth on her upper denture.

A front one - FFS!

She said it would look really unsightly and didn't want me to see her looking like that, which I could understand.

Anyway, she said she'd take it to get it repaired, and hopefully it would be okay for the weekend.

I packed my case as usual and put it in the car on Friday, as I was hoping she'd have it repaired by then.

She was having it fitted late in the afternoon.

It got to four thirty and she hadn't rung, so I set off down the M1 to London on the off chance.

I'd been driving about half an hour when Misty texted me, so I pulled into the first available service station and rang her back.

Unfortunately the new denture didn't fit properly, so she called the weekend off.

Think it's a gurly thing!

I drove home feeling very low.

It wasn't because of her teeth, and I could understand why didn't want me to see her like that.

But I had more important things on my mind then!

Saturday 2 June
A couple of weeks before, Misty had brought me a lovely silver toe ring with a little ruby heart mounted in the centre.

I have never taken it off and still wear it to this day.

So when I was in Lincoln on Saturday I went to see if I could find one for her. Luckily there was a craft market in town, and I found a lovely little toe ring that had two little pink hearts at the top.

I had to have it. I posted it to Misty so it arrived for Thursday the seventh of June, which was a day I dreaded.

I haven't mentioned this before, but despite all the lovely times we spent together, there was an evil cloud lurking in the background.

Tranny's life is always shit!

Misty always had a lovely sexy drawling Australian voice, but ever since I had met her it had been a little bit hoarse.

Very sexy in its own way.

Shortly before we met she'd been to see a doctor for a routine health check.

Her own doctor couldn't see her for some reason, so she'd had a word with her ex-wife, who was in the medical profession. She arranged to see the ex-wife's doctor as an alternative.

Misty's own doctor knew she had a slightly sexy rasp to her voice, but he just dismissed it and never did anything about it.

Pillock!

The other doctor was in a different category altogether.

She did all the usual checks, and everything was fine until she asked Misty about the voice.

Misty said it had been like that for a while, but as she had no pain or a sore throat she had never thought anything of it.

The doctor was having none of that!

She wanted her to get it checked by a specialist, and the date was:

Thursday the seventh of June

She'd told me about this a few weeks ago, but being the gurl she was (and a Leo to boot), she just played it all down.

Said it was probably just a small cyst.

No big deal!

Well, it concerned me a little. I loved the gurl!

I asked her if she had a sore throat, as you always associate those with something more severe.

She said she had no discomfort at all.

Misty was confident that it was nothing to worry about, so I didn't.

Still thought it was a fairy story with a happy ending?

I remember that Thursday very well. We were having those awful summer storms, and it rained all day and just seemed dark.

Like a bad omen!

I used to drive to Grantham, get the train to Leeds, and walk to the office. There'd been flooding everywhere, and we even had to change trains to get through to Leeds that morning.

Really shitty day in all ways!

Misty's appointment was in the afternoon, so I didn't expect her to ring until I finished work after four thirty.

I set off back to the station under black clouds and got there at about five. The train didn't leave for about twenty minutes, so I sat in a carriage and worried.

I just wished Misty would text me or ring me.

Just wanted to know she was okay, as I was sure she would be.

The phone suddenly rang. It was Misty.

I said hello and then waited.

"It's not good news, hun!"

She'd just come out of the hospital, where she'd been most of the afternoon, and was driving home.

Said we should speak tonight when I got home.

It felt like a very dark evening going home that night.

She rang me about seven thirty. The consultant had given her a full check and then put a camera down her throat. She had a growth near her vocal cords, and it was a tumour.

That was like a shell shock!

Misty had always brushed it off in the past, but now she told me she knew what it was before she went.

The only thing they didn't know was whether it was malignant or not.

They needed to do further tests for that.

Didn't speak much more.

Everything else seemed superfluous.

I arranged to see her on Friday.

<u>Friday 8 June</u>
I drove down to Misty's straight from work and got there at about half past eight, feeling shattered.

They'd started working on the bottom of the M1 and there were hold-ups. I was only about thirty miles from Misty, but it took at least an hour to get through.

Misty was dressed when I got there, and she gave me a large vodka and tonic and made some supper.

Must have drunk a bottle of wine with the meal.

One of those nights when booze has no effect.

We talked about anything and everything except what I really wanted to know.

There was no mention of the tests she'd had.

After supper I went upstairs to have a bath and got dressed.

When I came down we sat and cuddled each other. I broached the subject of the tests.

Misty said she didn't really want to talk about them, but I knew she did.

In the end she opened up!

She told me what the doctors had said - that they'd take a biopsy to check it out and then they'd laser it. All done and dusted.

Didn't sound that bad the way she told me.

We chatted a bit longer, and then Misty dropped another bombshell on me. She said she'd had a coronary a few years ago when she was on holiday with her father-in-law. She'd been driving a minibus in Ireland when it happened.

First I heard about that.

Then it got worse!

She went on to tell me that the consultant had referred her to an anaesthetist that same afternoon.

The reason for the referral was that she'd need a general anaesthetic for the biopsy, and given the previous heart attack they were worried about it.

As in could she survive it!

They didn't want any complications on the operating table and needed to find out what state her arteries were in.

She was booked for an angiogram.

Anyway, we talked about it all, as Misty just wanted to tell me and get it out of the way.

She made it sound like it was no big deal.

She laughed and said she'd lose her husky voice.

We sat up till well into the morning and both got a bit drunk and maybe a little melancholy.

Think we both wanted to forget about it all at that stage and pretend it was a bad dream.

On Saturday morning we both got up late, and Misty wanted to go into town. It must have been about one o'clock before we set off.

We dropped some things off at a dry cleaner and then looked for a place that was open.

It was about two thirty, and most places had closed, but there's always somewhere in London.

We found a little Italian restaurant and lazed away the afternoon.

Lots of ouzo and we got a bit smashed again!

In the evening we both decided to get dressed up to the nines.

I always did Misty's false eyelashes, as she could never manage them herself. She used to lie on the bed and Eddy always used to come and join in.

He thought it was a great game, as he got in the way.

I didn't really have a dress to suit the occasion, so Misty lent me her zebra dress and a spare long auburn wig.

It completely changed my image and made me look about ten years younger.

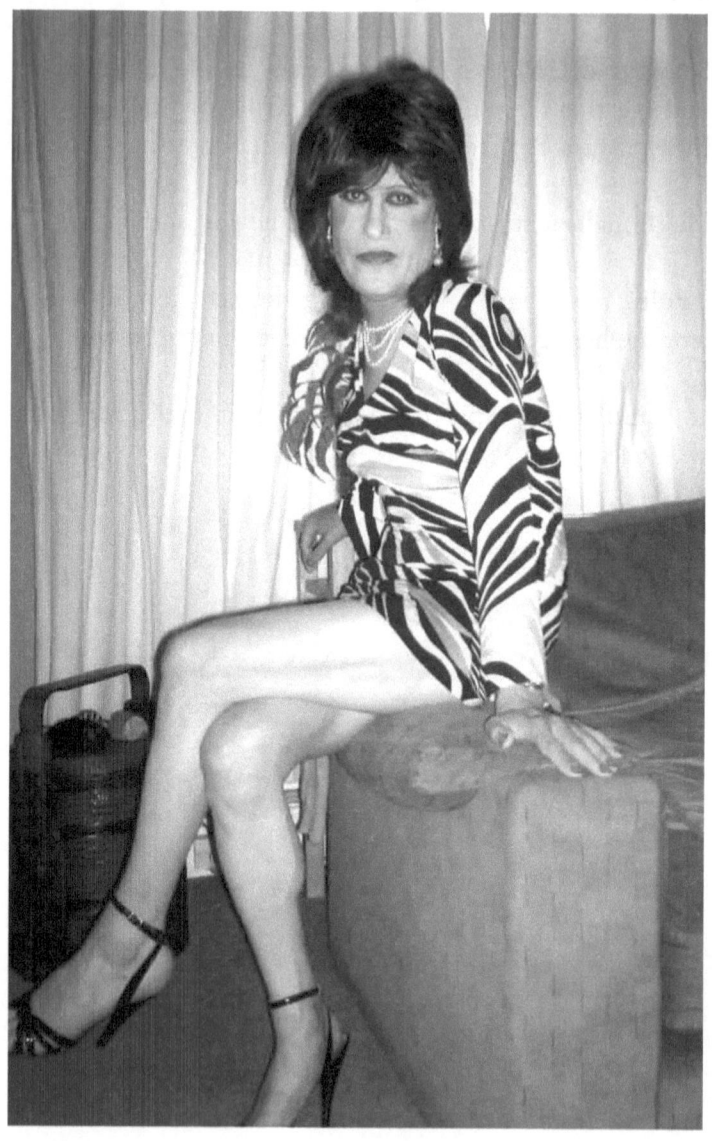

Misty was going to give me a ring that used to belong to Simone (RG), but I said no.

She'd been with Misty for about a year, and she was a beautiful Persian girl who was something of an artist. But she had a bad coke habit, and to cut a long story short she went berserk one day at Misty's.

Combination of coke and drink!

She fell in a drunken state in Misty's bath, and there was blood everywhere. That explained the cracked tiles round the bath.

She attacked Misty, who had to physically hold her down while she rang the police.

The police eventually took her away, and she ended being locked up and then sectioned.

It was only because she admitted it was all her fault that Misty didn't end up in prison for battering her.

I certainly didn't want her ring.

We stayed up late again that night and spent a lot of time cuddling. All the trouble seemed to disappear when we held each other tightly in bed.

Was a good night with my gurl.

<u>Friday 15 June</u>
I went down and it was just the two of us all weekend.

When I got there on Friday, Misty was in a much better mood than last weekend, and we didn't mention medical things at all.

Life went back to normal - well as normal as it can be for two old queens!

I sat and had a drink when I got there and noticed that Misty had printed off a picture of me from last weekend.

She'd framed it and placed in on the little table next to the light by the sofa.

Seemed to have an air of permanence.

I signed it with love.

"Tart with a heart!"

We had some supper and I got changed. Misty showed me her revamped Chix profile.

She'd put a note on it that said she was going to lose her husky voice as the doctors had found a little lump and were going to zap it with a laser.

Guess it was her way of turning it into a bit of a joke.

Bloody Aussie humour!

We went into town on Saturday, and I visited a chemist to buy something intimate.

Gurl has to be clean - LOL!

It was a big chemist that specialised in medical aids for both men and women.

Well, apparatus and stuff.

Anyway, I took the said item to the counter to pay, and the assistant told me very deliberately that what I was buying was for women.

I told him I knew.

Look on his face was indescribable!

I had my video camera that weekend, and we started making our first video, which was quite exciting. Well, very, when we watched it back!

Ready for my close-up now, Mr Deville!

Had loads of fun that night, and I've still got the video which I edited down to cut out the off scenes. There were quite a few of those which were quite funny. Somehow I didn't think they'd be appropriate to send to the "You've Been Framed" show.

I wore Misty's fur coat for most of it.

Lights, camera, action - tarts on film - LOL!

<u>Monday 18 June</u>

Misty rang me on the Monday evening before she went off to the Phily for dinner. Said she'd been listening to Chris Rea on the way and that a particular track reminded her of me. It was called *Giverny*. I still listen to it a lot, and it always reminds me of her.

The words might sound a bit corny but they summed up how we felt at the time:

> *"And in this strange and holy place*
> *I looked for love and found it everywhere"*

She said she wasn't playing and had just gone there for a chat. To be honest I wouldn't have minded even if she was playing.

I loved her a lot and knew she'd always play around, but hopefully she would always come back to me.

Someone else told me later "it was only sex," and I'd like to think that was right when Misty played with other gurlz. It always was with me.

It's who we are!

Not many of us are totally faithful to one gurl in body, but then I guess it's the mind that really counts in the long run.

She told me she was going for a further scan on her neck on Thursday, so I waited for her to call in the evening with the results.

Hope it wasn't any worse.

Thursday 21 June
Misty rang me in the evening.

There was nothing to report really, except they hadn't found anything else, which was good news.

It meant it was probably still localised to her throat. So the next step would be a full body scan to confirm this, and then a biopsy to check if it was malignant.

Saturday 23 June
Misty had been a bit concerned about all the driving I'd been doing, and to be honest it was tiring me out.

For a change she suggested we meet on Saturday at the Campanile and go to PP in the evening. The Campanile was a favourite tranny friendly hotel, although it had a lot of straight guests.

PP had started running another BNO night on the last Saturday night of the month, so we thought we'd see what it was like.

I felt a bit strange about not going down to see her on the Friday and wondered if something else was in the air, but it was just me being oversensitive as usual.

What we didn't realise was that because Sparkle was on in Manchester they cancelled the Saturday night, as most gurlz would be there.

Ooh, Sparkle!

Sparkle was an annual transvestite posing event with beauty pageants and discos at night.

A lot of people thought it was all fixed, which it was! If you looked at the winners each year they all seem to be connected to the industry in some way or another.

Not many places where a hooker gets first prize!

At the Campanile we wandered down to the restaurant, expecting it to be full of gurlz.

What a shock we had!

The restaurant was nearly empty except for a few straight couples and the odd family. I felt a bit nervous, but Misty was so full of confidence she just treated it as normal.

When we sat down we were next to a family and had some funny looks from the little children. You can imagine them asking their parents what two men were doing wearing dresses, and the parents reply.

"Going to a fancy dress party so just eat your dinner."

In truth it was just like sitting in a restaurant like normal people. No one batted an eyelid. There may have been some whispered conversations from the children but nothing else.

After dinner we trotted off to PP and went to the bar upstairs. There were hardly any gurlz there, and we soon found out that the BNO had been cancelled due to Sparkle.

It didn't make much difference to us. We sat chatting and were fairly oblivious to the rest of the people there. Misty took her camera and had someone take a picture of us.

When we'd had enough we went back to the hotel. You can guess the rest. I can still recall exactly what happened, which I not about to repeat. Afterwards we just curled up and went to sleep in each other's arms.

Nothing had changed - was just me being stupid.

We left on Sunday morning at about eleven. I remember us going down to the cars with our luggage before we each drove off in separate directions.

I felt very sad as I watched Misty go.

We'd only spent one night together, and I guess I did feel cheated in a way. I was so used to spending two nights with her.

I know nothing had changed, but as I drove home I did just wonder a little.

I was feeling bad about that, and I was worried as I knew that next week she'd have to go off for a full body scan.

They wanted to check that it hadn't spread anywhere.

Misty went to the hospital for a full scan and rang me in the evening to tell me about it.

She didn't think she'd need to take her shoes off, so she'd kept her nail varnish on her toes. She had beautiful long purple toenails, and toe rings, including the one I'd given her.

The nurses showed her into the room with the scanner and asked her to strip right down and put a smock on.

When they said strip off, they meant it!

I think the nurses, who had seen it all before, had a little giggle. But Misty told me they really admired her nails and when she'd finished her scan even asked her where they could get similar toe rings.

Misty said she wasn't sure, as the one she had on was a present from her girlfriend.

Little old me!

She got the results of the scan a few days later on the Thursday, which was good news. The doctors had told her it was only local and restricted to her throat.

She was very up about it!

<u>Friday 22 June to Sunday 8 July</u>
Over the next few weeks I went to see her every weekend, and I guess life returned to near normality.

We just enjoyed each other's company. She was still awaiting the biopsy, but for the time being we forgot about that most of the time.

Nothing had changed on the medical front, and I guess we both buried our heads in the sand. We had some wonderful weekends together and during that time saw no one else. To all intents and purpose we were just like a married couple.

Well two old trannies!

My contract had finished, and I was starting a new to job in mid July. I used to go down early on a Friday and get there mid afternoon.

I used to get to the end of the M1 and then go to big Tesco store at Brentwood to buy a bottle of wine and some flowers, as I knew Misty really liked them. Lillies were her favourite.

Misty was working for herself and had taken over the property next door and turned it into an office.

She usually made sure she finished early and told her personal assistant she could go early as well.

I remember we spent a few late afternoons on Fridays sitting in the sun on the back terrace, drinking vodka and tonics and just enjoying being together, knowing we had the whole weekend to look forward to.

The back door was always open, and Eddy used to keep disappearing off to see his lady friend, a lovely little white cat from a few doors away. Think she was a bit disappointed.

Little guy had been done!

Fridays were usually quite late nights, so we'd get up late on Saturdays and go to Tesco or sometimes straight into London, have a look round the shops, and maybe some lunch.

If we went to town Misty would pick up some cigarettes from a little Asian guy who sold them from under the counter, as they had been smuggled in and were about half the price.

We used to go to some nice restaurants, and Misty paid for it all, saying she was putting it down as business expenses.

I asked Misty about smoking, and she told me some porkies at the time. She said her growth had nothing to do with it. The doctors had told her it wasn't related, which of course it was.

She had a brother in Australia who was a surgeon specialising in laser treatment. She had a good long talk with him, and according to her he'd told her it would do more harm than good to give up now.

Well, I believed anything at that time.

If we didn't go to town we'd get some provisions from Tesco and have a barbeque on the back terrace.

I used to get quite tired so had a sleep on Saturday afternoons while Misty watched cricket or sat on the back terrace drinking.

It was a glorious time, and I guess we were very much in love.

Tranny love - LOL!

The weather in London was brilliant, and we just enjoyed each other's company. Everything felt just right.

There was the odd conversation about medical matters, but in those weeks we pretended they'd go away and life would go on the way it was.

Neither of us thought seriously about the future.

Too perfect for anything to spoil it!

I never took my bag home, and it stayed in Misty's spare bedroom. It seemed that was where it should be, as I wasn't going to be dressing for anyone else.

I left everything there, including my toothbrush.

At the start of those weeks Misty had got me a key cut so I could let myself in if she was out and organise the parking tickets myself.

Just a "normal" couple!

<u>Friday 13 to Sunday 15 July</u>
We talked all week before I went down at the weekend, and Misty said she wanted to go to BNO.

We got dressed and sat and had a few glasses of wine, but it was getting late and eventually we decided not to go.

They'd introduced a smoking ban, and it would take us a good hour to get there, so we stayed in.

I must admit I was quite pleased, as I still didn't know what would happen, and any time we spent together was a bonus.

Instead we planned to go to the Philly on Saturday, but when we spoke again on Saturday morning neither of us was too keen.

We decided to go into town that day. We popped into Ann Summers, where Misty bought a little blue dolphin for me.

Not showing you a picture of that!

When we got back in the afternoon I was tired so had a small sleep with Eddy. It was a lovely sunny day, so Misty sat outside on the small patio having a few drinks and fell asleep in the sun.

Everything just felt right, and each weekend it was like coming home. I sensed that this weekend Misty really wanted to spend some time with just the both of us.

Sixth sense, I guess!

We got dressed later in the evening and took some lovely pictures featuring the blue dolphin on me.

Then we made a video, which was a bit naughty but very personal.

That evening when we went to bed Misty felt quite down. Normally it was me who ended up getting a cuddle, which I loved.

But today it was different.

We both got undressed, and I just sensed something. I turned over, gave her a cuddle, and held her tight as she drifted off to sleep.

She didn't say anything. There was no need to.

She was taller and stronger than me, but that night I knew she needed me to be strong.

I was holding a very frightened little gurl in my hands. Think the reality of it all was starting to bite.

I woke up on Sunday morning with the sun streaming in through the window. I really needed her to give me a cuddle, but she'd gone.

Misty had gone downstairs to make some coffee, and I was left alone, feeling a bit vulnerable.

I needed some reassurance from my gurl to tell me it would all be okay.

How would she know?

I knew it was all spinning through her head now.

I drove home on Sunday and spoke to Misty on Yahoo! in the evening, which was unusual.

She was very down and said she had mounting problems.

Not much I could say in reply!

She told me I was all she had in her life at the moment.

Good job it was on Yahoo!. I got so upset at hearing that I ended up in tears.

Not going to be easy, this!

I had started a new job in Peterborough, and on the Friday I drove down see Misty. I got there at about seven fifteen.

Misty was partially dressed and seemed in a lot better mood. She suggested we go to the Phily for dinner.

I was in two minds, as it was getting closer and closer to her biopsy. I really just wanted to spend as much time as I could with her.

Anyway, I knew she wanted to go, and most of all I wanted to see her enjoy herself. So I said okay and went to get changed quickly.

When I came downstairs she was having a drink and rolling a few joints. I don't know why I said it, but I did.

I looked at the drink and told her that if she wasn't careful she'd end up getting stopped by the police.

She used to drink a fair bit and always told me that she adopted the continental approach to drinking and driving, which I guess was "let's not worry about it right now."

As soon as I said that she stood in front of me, held her hands out, and smiled at me.

It was her way. She came back with the usual response and shrug of the shoulders as she took another drink.

"Had I ever seen her driving erratically or unsafely?"

I mentioned it was other idiots she had to watch out for.

She laughed, shrugged her shoulders again, and said I was a typical Capricorn.

Then she gave me one of those luscious, naughty looks that always melted me, and I knew we were going.

It was already about nine, so she went off the get the car and bring it round so I could climb in.

It was still quite hot, but I insisted on wearing her lovely fur coat as it felt so nice.

Probably just as well, as I would need it later!

We got to the Philly and she parked the car as usual, and we went down to the bar for a few quick drinks before dinner.

That was followed by a lovely meal with loads of wine, and then back down to the bar, where we had a few more whiskies.

You know what's coming now!

It was about one o'clock, and when we got outside the cold night air hit me. I felt quite tipsy and a little bit dreamy.

Misty fetched the car, so I got in and snuggled up beside her.

She lit a joint and drove off - LOL!

I asked her to put some music on, and as we drifted through London I thought how nice it would be to get home.

I just wanted us to go to bed, holding each other tight, as we drifted off to sleep.

After about fifteen minutes Misty pulled the car in.

I thought she wanted something out of the boot. Probably cigarettes, which she kept there.

Then she said those immortal words which I'll never forget.

"We're in trouble now."

I could tell from her voice that it was something serious. Suddenly I sat up and looked behind the car as Misty opened the door to step out.

Big blue flashing light!

Misty was ushered to the pavement, and I got out to see what was happening. She was told she'd been stopped as she was driving erratically.

Well, we knew that was complete nonsense.

I knew she was over the limit, but I'd seen her drive like this loads of times. The real truth was that they'd seen us dressed and knew we were a couple of TVs and decided they'd have some fun.

One young policeman brought out a breathalyser and told Misty to blow in it. She told him she couldn't due to the problem with her throat. Well, he wasn't buying that, and I could tell he was starting to get annoyed.

It didn't help that Misty was quite tall and towered over him. He told her she was now obstructing the course of justice and gave her a final chance. Misty protested again and said she couldn't, and that was it.

No more messing anymore!

The officer brought out some heavy cuffs and snapped them on her wrists. She was arrested and given a caution as they marched her to the back of the van.

She was going back to the station.

As she stood by the back of the van, another officer said he'd move the car and asked if there was anything either of us wanted before he drove it away.

I got Misty's male loafers and passed them to one officer who was going in the van.

This took a few minutes, and we both protested about the cuffs. This seemed very heavy-handed under the circumstances. The young officer who'd put them on relented and took them off.

It was just so stupid to have those on, and when he'd taken them off her wrists were bleeding quite badly.

At this point they drove the car away and Misty was put in the back of the van. I asked if I could go along with her, but the officers said no.

They told me I'd have to make my own way to wherever I was going. All they said was they were taking her to Paddington Green.

Misty was in some shock and said nothing at the time. She assumed I'd taken the house keys from the car and was going to make my way home, but I hadn't known the keys were there.

Before I knew it they all had gone!

Suddenly I was alone in a deserted street in the middle of London. It was about two o'clock in the morning, and all I had on me was about seven pounds.

I'd spent most of the rest of it on drinks at the Phily.

I wasn't going to get far at this time of night. I couldn't have gone to Misty's even if I wanted to as I had no key, but in truth that didn't matter.

All I really wanted to do was go and see that Misty was okay. I decided I'd make my way to the station by some means or another.

First thing I did was sit on the pavement between two parked cars and take my 5-inch heels off. I knew I'd be walking, and they were already starting to kill me.

I remembered the direction the van had gone, so I set off that way. I was barefoot, with my heels in one hand and my handbag slung over my shoulder.

After about fifteen minutes I came to what looked like a taxi stand in the middle of a wide street. I stood there and waited for one to appear.

It really didn't matter to me that I was dressed. I didn't even give it a second thought. All I wanted was to see Misty.

I must have been there for about half an hour, and most of the taxis I flagged had passengers and just kept going by. Eventually a private one stopped.

I asked how far Paddington Green was, and he said I should walk as it was just around the corner. But I persuaded him to give me a lift.

Think it cost a fiver, which was good, as that only left with me with two pounds.

The police station was high security and had a big rotating signpost that said Scotland Yard. The entrance was up some granite steps, and at that time of night it all looked a bit foreboding.

I walked up the steps and into the reception area, which was completely empty. Not a soul about, so I rang the bell on the desk and about ten minutes later a girl turned up.

She really looked like she cared (not) - LOL!

I told her why I was there, and she said Misty was being held until the duty solicitor turned up. Said it could be some hours, but it all depended on him.

Misty could be held till Monday morning - FFS!

Well, all I could do was sit and wait. There were horrible plastic chairs which were as hard as nails, and bolted to the floor. As I was the only one there I tucked my legs up and tried to sleep.

I dozed a little on and off, but after an hour or so I was desperate for some relief and had a look round for the public toilettes. There were none, and I really had to go.

I had no option but to nip outside and duck down under the steps. Kept thinking there must be CCTV cameras about and they would catch it on film and I'd end up getting booked.

That would look embarrassing at work. Tranny caught outside Paddington Green Police Station and booked for doing you know what (allegedly). Didn't think that would go down too well with the management at work!

The police station was quite close to a hostel, and round about four o'clock the idiots started trooping in. As only I was there I became the immediate target for them.

It wasn't because I was dressed!

That didn't seem to bother them in the slightest. All they wanted was a captive audience.

I can't remember what they said, as I just nodded in agreement to it all. It was the usual political ranting and raving about how unfair the system was.

One guy began to get quite irate, and I could feel a fight coming on. I managed to calm the situation but could tell it would soon get out of hand.

He was getting ready to lamp someone - Me!

Fortunately for me, his attention was distracted at just the right time by other events. It was about five o'clock and the door behind reception opened, and there were two police officers and Misty!

She was pretty glad to get out of there, and I was equally pleased to see some officers. It saved me from getting a pasting.

What was going on in the cells was a lot worse than what I'd had to put up with. Let's just say the cells were fully packed with yardies and other miscreants who haunted London at night, and they weren't overly keen on TVs.

We didn't hang around, and once she'd been given the address of her car we left sharpish.

The car was some distance away so we decided to get a taxi. Now, getting a taxi from the Philly and back is easy.

This wasn't!

It was about half five in the morning, so most taxis were off duty. She had loafers on, and I had no heels. Our makeup looked well past its best, and we were both obviously TV gurlz. Trying to persuade a cab to stop was nigh impossible.

We waited by some traffic lights, as that meant anyone who came by had to slow down. Each driver took one look at us and disappeared quickly once he knew what we were.

They weren't taking any chances!

Finally one had to stop at the lights, and he had his passenger window down. Misty had a conversation with him, but he was thinking twice about it and was just about to drive off. Misty told him she needed to a lift to pick up her car.

Said it was a Saab convertible.

That seemed to swing it, and we both jumped in very gratefully. The cab driver found the right street and dropped us off. It was a huge road with cars parked down each side as far as the eye could see.

We walked up and down it for ages and still couldn't find the car. Misty thought it might be up a side street, so we walked up there and finally found it.

Thank God!

It felt such a relief to sit in the car and head off back to Misty's as the sun begun to come up. She said she had waited an hour and a half for the duty solicitor to turn up, and they still hadn't taken a blood sample. She'd thought I'd gone home but was very grateful I'd waited for her.

Well, I had to. It was only right.

When we got back to Misty's it must have been almost six in the morning. We both sat there feeling like we'd been dragged though a hedge backwards.

What a night that was!

Despite how tired we were, we were also so full of energy that neither of us could sleep.

We had some coffee and very large whiskies, and then I got the video camera out.

Funny how something like that can make you so excited. We made a great video. It was electric and very highly charged.

By eight o'clock both of us were ready to fall over, so we ended up in bed and fell asleep till at least midday.

We both woke up and were still so hyper that we got intimate again. Then we fell asleep till two.

We talked about the previous night, and Misty said if the worst came to the worst she'd apply for an Australian licence.

Said she knew someone else who'd lost his licence and had done it.

I couldn't see it really and think it was wishful thinking on her behalf.

She still needed her car for her business, and there was no way she was using public transport.

"I'm not that sort of gurl, sweetie."

The rest of Saturday was a blur. I had a massive hangover, but we still got dressed and had a few drinks before going to bed early for a proper night's sleep.

I drove back on Sunday feeling like death warmed up, just needing my bed again.

My son asked how the weekend was, and I just said fine.

Some things are better kept secret.

<u>Tuesday 24 July</u>
Misty had been for another test and also to see the heart specialist and anaesthetist. They said she would need a general anaesthetic for the biopsy.

Not good news!

We chatted on Yahoo! and Misty said the heart specialist was quite concerned about her blocked arteries from the coronary a few years ago. She was even talking about the possibility of a bypass before the biopsy could take place.

Suddenly I had a terrible thought that hadn't occurred to me till now!

Whether she had the bypass or the biopsy, she'd need a general for either.

She could still die on the operating table from either of those!

FFS!

I didn't say anything.

She didn't want to talk about it and basically said her life was now in the hands of the surgeons.

We changed the subject and made arrangements for the weekend for me to go and see her on Friday.

<u>Friday 27 to Sunday 29 July</u>
I drove down on the Friday. Not sure what happened that night, but I know I had too much to drink. Despite that we made another video.

Misty's birthday was on the Sunday. I knew I had to drive back on Sunday morning so on the Friday I gave her a little leopard skin pendant on a gold chain.

On Saturday we went into town again and stopped at one of those real burger places for lunch. In the afternoon I had another sleep with Eddy while Misty watched cricket. Then in the evening we got dressed again and made another video.

As we were making them with no cameraman, it sometimes took a good few sessions before we could put them all together to make something decent.

Misty made some breakfast on Sunday morning before I left, which was something she'd never done before. Anyway after breakfast she took the plates and put them in the dishwasher, which she switched on. That was a big mistake. She used to hide her pot in there and didn't remember till it was too late so she had to dry it all out again.

Apart from that there was nothing very special about the weekend in terms of what we did, but then there didn't need to be.

It just felt right spending time together.

She told me she was off to court on Tuesday morning to have a hearing about the driving licence.

<u>Tuesday 31 July</u>
I rang Misty at lunchtime to see how the court case had gone. She told me it had been adjourned until the twenty-eighth of August.

I could tell she wasn't happy, as the case was now postponed, and there was no news on the medical front either.

Everything just seemed up in the air.

Misty rang me in the evening to say she was going out to dinner and that she wasn't playing around.

I loved her a lot by this time, and I wouldn't have cared if she did at that stage.

I told her to be careful driving, but I knew it fell on deaf ears and she'd be well over the limit.

She reckoned that if she'd only been pulled once in three-odd years, then the chances of her getting pulled again were minimal.

I sat at home thinking of her at the Phily and just wished I could have been there.

I wasn't sure where all this was heading, but something unsettled me. I just wanted it to last as long as it could.

<u>Friday 3 to Sunday 5 August</u>

I drove down to Misty's on the Friday, and we did the usual. Had a chat about the previous week, had a meal, and then I had a bath and got dressed.

It was all becoming a bit of a very pleasant routine, and I lived for the weekends.

On Saturday Misty had arranged for a cameraman to come over, but I was in two minds about it. Misty said she'd spoken to him on Yahoo! and said he was reliable, so I agreed.

He was supposed to text to confirm he was coming in the late afternoon, but he never did.

Misty texted him and told him he'd blown it.

Admirers didn't get a second chance, but Misty was determined to play that weekend, so she had a look to see who else was about.

We spoke to Oudie, who was in London with his family. Oudie was a Saudi prince who had been threatening to come over for ages.

He had some pictures on the website, and we knew he was the real deal, but unreliable.

Misty blew him out in the end and told him not to bother again!

Misty had another look on the website to see who she could come up with. She found Valerie, who lived in Braintree.

She didn't drive, so the taxi just to get her here was going to cost her 50 pounds. She arranged to come at eight thirty and also wanted help with her makeup.

Nine o'clock came round and Valerie still hadn't arrived. She rang us and said she was over the other side of London and that the taxi driver didn't know where he was.

Misty gave him some directions, but she was getting really fed up with it. I was starting to wonder about what the evening held after all this.

Valerie eventually turned up at about ten thirty. She hadn't been out much and sat there chattering away through nerves when she arrived.

I took her upstairs and did her makeup, and we took some pictures of her.

It was so late by then that I was not in the mood for playing, so eventually Misty and I made some excuse and went upstairs to bed and fell asleep.

We left Valerie downstairs with a duvet.

We woke in the morning and I guess having someone else there had an effect on Misty.

It was raw unbridled passion!

I told Misty to close the door in case Valerie came up, but Misty didn't care. I made a bit of noise, and Valerie must have heard it, as I saw a figure standing over us. Valerie tried to join in, but in all honesty it was as if she wasn't there.

Neither of us paid her any attention.

Misty satisfied herself, and I was in pure heaven.

We hadn't invited Valerie to join us, so when we were spent we stopped. I guess Valerie standing there also killed the passion!

I decided I ought to get changed as I'd have to go soon, and Misty went down to make some coffee.

We left Valerie on the bed and sorted ourselves out.

I got changed in the spare room. When I'd finished I went down to join Misty and as I walked past the main bedroom I saw Valerie was asleep on the bed and I couldn't wake her.

She was dead to the world.

It took ages to sort her out and get her downstairs. She could hardly walk.

Turns out she'd been up most of the night watching our videos and had polished of a bottle of whiskey.

I poured some coffee down her neck to try and wake her up.

Misty let me sort Valerie out, as she wasn't too good at that sort of thing, but she ordered her a taxi.

I had to virtually pour her into that and tell the driver where to take her.

It was a huge relief when she finally went away.

Shortly after, it was time for me to go.

I drove back feeling very dejected, as I really didn't know how much longer Misty and I would have.

Saturday night had been such as waste of time!

<u>Friday 10 to Sunday 12 August</u>
I got down after work on the Friday and got dressed as usual. We had a lovely time that night.

Misty had been speaking to another gurl during the week and had arranged for her to come over on the Saturday. She asked me what I thought about it.

I didn't really want another gurl there, but I knew Misty did, so I said yes. Guess it helped Misty take her mind off things.

With everything going on at present we seemed to be living on somewhat of a knife edge, and I never knew what was round the corner.

Just got jealous of sharing!

Anyway, we arranged it and spent ages getting ready on the Saturday night before Sally arrived. She turned up at about eight thirty and was quite well-spoken and brought a few bottles with her.

Well, she got dressed and came down to join us, and we did the usual chit chat thing.

I wasn't sure what Sally did, but we got the impression she was quiet high up in the Ministry of Defence.

Secret squirrel stuff again!

Misty and Sally smoked quite a lot of pot and got really stoned, and then Misty got quite cross with me.

She'd never done that before.

Couldn't understand what was happening.

Then she started taking the mickey out of me. I could feel something was in the air and didn't know what to do. Just ended up pissed.

We did play a bit, but Sally was a very strange gurl who was obsessed with making it all last as long as possible.

More mechanical than anything else.

There was no passion there at all - often the way with some TVs !

It was a weird night. Sally had only shaved partially and wore two corsets, even in bed!

I felt really rough on Sunday morning, so I went downstairs still dressed to make some coffee and have a cigarette. Sally was upstairs getting changed. I was on the sofa as Misty came down looking bloody awful.

She looked so depressed.

She said she really needed to apologise to Sally about last night and that she needed to re-evaluate her life and where she was going.

My heart just sank when I heard that. I just sat there and listened.

She looked so distant from me, and it was like I wasn't there.

It could only mean it was the end for me.

I babbled some stupid excuse and went back upstairs to change. I know I had tears welling in my eyes.

Couldn't believe it was over.

I went into the spare room where my clothes were and sat on the floor and cried and cried. Sally was so wrapped up in what she was doing that I don't think she even noticed. I went and cleared everything out of the bathroom and packed all that into my bag.

Felt so final.

I had one last look around before taking my things down. I knew I wouldn't be coming back to that bed.

Or even the house!

I just felt totally numb.

I was like a blank canvas, with all the life squeezed out of me.

Took my suitcase down and Misty said nothing about it, so it I knew it was over. Misty asked me to stay till Sally had gone.

I knew a farewell speech was coming, so I made a coffee and sat silently till Sally came down and said her farewells. Misty apologised to Sally about the night, and then she left.

I wanted the Earth to swallow me and I sat there in floods of tears waiting for Misty to say a final goodbye to me.

Misty repeated what she had said before. She needed to re-evaluate her life. But then she added:

It didn't include me!

Said she was a one-woman gurl, which was why she needed to apologise to Sally.

I couldn't believe what she was saying. I'd gotten it all so wrong and misread all the signs.

My tears turned to joy. We sat and cuddled with such passion as we held each other so tight. I could feel tremors running though both of our bodies.

I wasn't dressed, but that didn't seem to matter to either of us.

We went back upstairs, and being honest, Misty took me there and then on the bed.

Never known love like that!

Time had moved on, and I needed to get back home, so I took my suitcase back upstairs. We had another coffee before I knew I had to go.

I still couldn't stop crying, as it was all a bit overwhelming.

I drove home feeling on top of the world!

Very happy TV - LOL!

<u>Tuesday 14 August</u>
I didn't speak to Misty on the Sunday or Monday, but I sent her a couple of texts and we arranged to speak on Tuesday evening.

I was having problems with my laptop and couldn't connect to Yahoo! for about thirty minutes that night. Misty sent me a text asking where I was.

I sent her a text back to say I was home and should be online soon. I got connected at about nine and asked her the inevitable question.

Was there any progress on the medical front?

She said the surgery was booked for next week but that it might not happen. Apparently the consultant, doctor, and anaesthetist still had to finalise things.

Misty got a bit frustrated, as she didn't think I was listening or following the conversation.

But I was and I understood everything!

She said she thought they'd put her in the box marked "too hard to handle".

No one seemed to want to take responsibility for the outcomes if anything went wrong.

She was very down and said she could end up dying on the table or just carry on with the way her throat was.

Great choice, she said!

She knew everything was looming up ahead of her.

Everything seemed to have gone wrong!

I loved her so much, and now it looked like she might be taken away from me. We had an understanding now, and I couldn't believe that next weekend might be our last.

I told Misty I'd take the following Friday off and come down to her. Misty was talking about the next bank holiday and us spending three days together, and I said I'd arrange to take the Friday off for that too. In the scheme of things it seemed like a long way off, and with so much happening in Misty's life it might not happen.

Not sure what it was, but something deep inside told me our fragile world wouldn't last much longer.

I don't know why, but I had this sixth sense that it wouldn't end in us falling out in a whimper, but in Misty's death.

I was crying at the other end!

<u>Friday 17 to Sunday 19 August</u>
I got to Misty's at about five as I had the day off work.
We chatted and the inevitable question came up.

Misty told me she had an appointment for the biopsy
next week, but she knew it wouldn't happen as they still
hadn't made their minds up.

She didn't bother dressing as she wasn't in the mood.

Nothing else to report that weekend.

<u>Wednesday 22 August</u>
For some reason I felt low all day, but as I drove home
Misty texted me, which cheered me up to no end.

She'd spoken to a solicitor, who told her that she'd need
evidence for the trial.

No one had told her that it was her responsibility to
collect it, and the trial was next Tuesday. It didn't leave
much time to get anything sorted.

She also said she wanted to go to the Phily on Saturday.

I was a bit hesitant about her driving again, but she
insisted, as she didn't think she'd get stopped again.

Typical Misty - LOL!

<u>Saturday 25 to Monday 27 August</u>
As it was a bank holiday on the Monday I drove down on the Saturday instead of the Friday. All the driving was making me tired, so spending an extra night at home probably made sense. I arrived at about twelve and got dressed early.

After twisting Misty's arm we ended up going in a taxi on the basis that I paid for the journey there.

Misty rang up a local taxi firm and they sent round some old Irish guy. Well, he pulled up right outside the house and even opened the door for us both.

Being treated like real gurlz!

He knew exactly what we were but just chatted away like he thought nothing of it. When we got there he did the same again.

Bless him.

It was a sunny evening, so when we got to the Philly we went downstairs for a drink and then out into the garden.

We met some married gay guys out there who were outrageous but really good company.

Pissed as farts!

The bride was a very thin little wiry guy in jeans and a tee shirt and Dr Martens boots. He smoked a dainty little enamelled pipe.

The groom, on the other hand, was a big jolly chap with a huge ring through his nose and one big nipple pin. He wore Dr Martens boots like his partner and an outrageous red PVC kilt with shoulder straps and a little black leather waistcoat.

He was court clerk!

They'd both been to the races that day and were well oiled but were still quaffing champagne.

We couldn't get a table in the restaurant as it was too busy. Jade gave us a table outside on the verandah, which overlooked the gay guys in the garden.

I knew they were ogling me, so I flashed my legs and really played up to them. After having dinner we ended up back in the garden with them and had a real laugh.

Kathy came in a bit later. She was a film producer and a dom who had her own dungeon and collected subs.

Misty had never seen eye to eye with her, but this evening it was all "darling" this and "darling" that!

Misty and me at the Phily

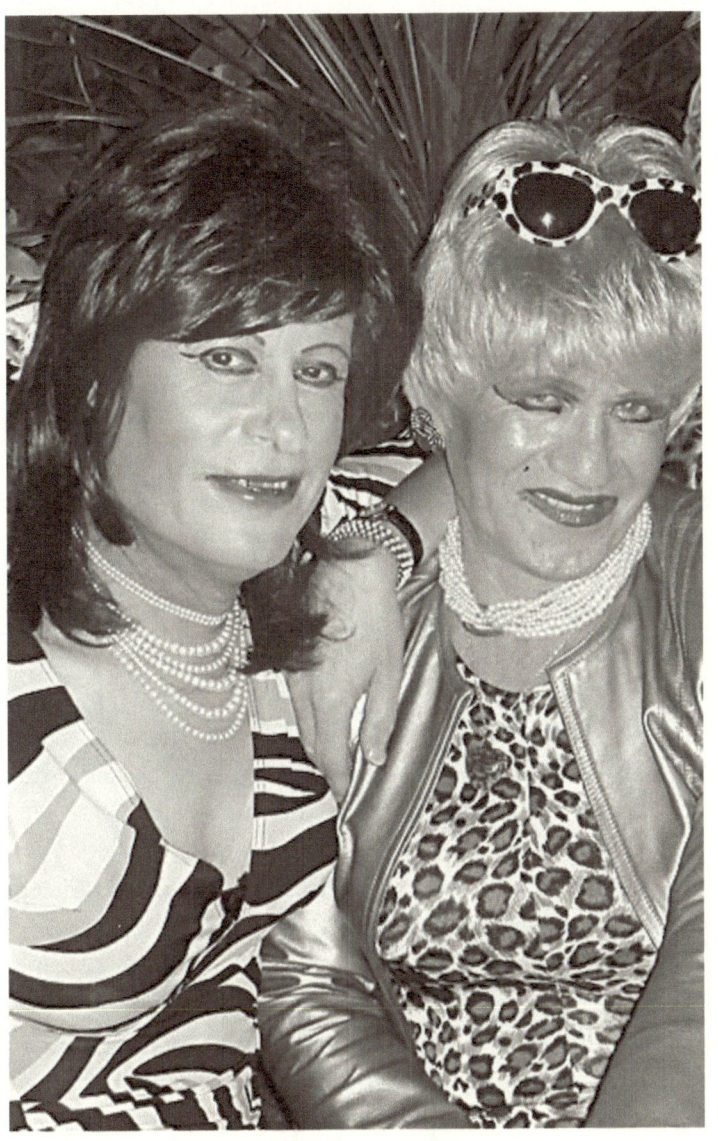

The gay guys ended up taking all of our pictures.

I ended up getting really pissed. When it was closing time Misty sat me in a chair under the red canopy as she ordered a taxi. She had to help me into the taxi, and I collapsed with my head in her lap.

I really don't remember how we got into the house, but somehow I got undressed and crashed out in bed.

Believe it or not, I felt fine on Sunday morning and very frisky, so we did -LOL! Neither of us was dressed, and it just felt so natural.

I didn't have to drive back till the Monday so we had a great time just being together on the rest of Sunday.

Tuesday 28 August
Misty's court case was today, so I rang her after work.

She'd been there most of the day only to find out that it was postponed until the second of October. Gave her the opportunity to get some new evidence.

She was going to see a lung specialist to get some written confirmation that she couldn't do a breathalyser.

I said, "Won't the specialist be suspicious and think you're pulling a flanker?" You wouldn't have to be a genius to put two and two together. Misty's reply was that she was a good actor!

I spoke to Misty on the phone in the evening to see if she'd made any progress on the medical front, but there was no news.

I was having trouble with my teeth, and Misty suggested I borrow some of her amoxicillin. She'd had a lot of dental trouble in the past, and the ex-wife had given her a supply. In fact her bathroom cabinet looked a little like a small chemist's.

She was always big on self-prescribing. I remember she once told me that she picked up something very nasty in Hong Kong at a Cathouse. A Chinese guy took her to a local chemist, and she got one enormous black pill that cleared it all up in twenty-four hours.

She told me she was waking up with a sore throat each morning, which really worried me.

It had been at least three months since she was first diagnosed with the tumour, and no progress had been made on any front.

Misty had been in contact with Frankie, an old friend who lived in America. She would be in England this weekend.

Misty had arranged for her to meet us on the Saturday if I was okay with it.

<u>Friday 31 August to Sunday 2 September</u>
I went down on the Friday, and we had a glorious time just dressing and being together.

We made another video to complete our collection. Misty wanted me to combine it with the others, as she wanted to show it to Frankie on Saturday.

Frankie came over on the Saturday night, and although I'd never met her before I took to her straight away.

She was a really nice gurl who dressed extremely well, in very expensive clothes. She brought a couple of bottles of wine, and we sat and chatted in the lounge for a while and got acquainted.

Misty cooked a Burmese curry, and we all we sat round the kitchen table and had dinner while Frankie relayed some of her stories.

It was all a bit incongruous, really.

She was an antique arms dealer who had come across the pond in order to bid on some pieces she could sell in the fairs in the US. This time she had won forty Vickers machine guns.

As you can imagine, that meant she had a military background.

Ex-SAS - close combat specialist!

She could only be described as having an extremely colourful past, and I wouldn't have wanted to be someone who picked a fight with her just because she had a dress on.

But in femme form Frankie was a very gentle and loving creature.

Every inch a real lady - LOL!

What I found out at dinner made me ever so grateful we shared the same lifestyle.

Would not have liked to be taken prisoner by her!

She told us that one occasion they needed to make some prisoners talk so they took the three of them up in a helicopter. Well one was pushed out the door and the others lost control of a few bodily functions and told them everything. At this point the others were then given the boot out of the door. Still on balance I'd have probably preferred that to being flayed to the bone and then being boiled alive which was another alternative.

You might be surprised at the number of Armed forces that are gurls!

After supper we watched a few of our videos, played a bit, and generally had a really nice time.

We both asked her if she wanted to stay the night, but at about two o'clock she went back to her camper van, which was parked a few streets away.

Misty and I just sat and had a drink before going to bed. She told me played in Frankie's van a few times outside the Phily which made me laugh. I can just imagine the van rocking!

For the next few weeks I went down every weekend.

Driving straight from work on the Friday and staying there till Sunday morning had now become a regular event. We made some more videos, which were getting quite good at now.

This was a day I had really been dreading.

Misty was due for her biopsy!

She'd rung me on the Monday to say she had to be there at seven thirty in the morning and she couldn't eat or drink after ten at night. I wished her luck and sent her a good luck text on the Tuesday morning.

All I could do was sit and wait for news!

She rang me at about eight at night and was home by then. She'd been asleep for the operation, as they'd given her a general anaesthesia in the end.

She told me it had given her a slight sore throat but otherwise she was okay. Instead of going home she went to the Marylebone Cricketers Club and had a few drinks with some old cronies there.

That was typical Misty.

A few of the staff there knew she had a few darker secrets, but they kept it to themselves.

Wouldn't really do to broadcast that the team captain was a raging TV!

<u>Friday 21 to Sunday 22 September</u>
I drove down from work, and Misty said she wanted to throw a party on Saturday, as Frankie was in Britain and could come over. Misty invited Simone over, as she still fancied her and said she owed her one.

Simone turned up after the three of us had dinner, but it was an absolute disaster. She never stopped talking about her second hand Masseratii and what it did to the gallon. She used to be in a popular rock band so she wasn't short of a bob or two. Then she got onto her personal problems. She was convinced a Persian girl was stalking her. In the end no one else could get a word in edgeways.

Well, after an hour or so of that the rest of us knew there would be no party that night.

No one was in the mood, and she just killed the atmosphere stone-dead. Frankie made her excuses to leave at about three in the morning and nipped upstairs to the loo. I had a quick word with her and tried to persuade her to stop the night, but she didn't.

Simone left about the same time, and Misty and I just cuddled up together. Misty said Simone had changed. She'd put on a lot of weight and was obsessed with herself. Think that put Misty off, despite Simone's various attributes!

I know Simone rang Misty a few days later to apologise, as she knew she'd wrecked the night.

Waste of space!

<u>Wednesday 26 September</u>
Misty got the results of her biopsy.

I must admit that it had totally slipped my mind that day. Not sure if it was work or just because I had assumed everything would be okay and shut it ought of my mind.

I was driving home that night and got a text message from Misty, so I pulled over to read it.

All it said was, "It's not good news!"

I rang her straight away and she said it was a malignant growth. Still in the early stages, but they couldn't laser it, as it was too close to her voice box.

Throat cancer!!!

My heart sank when I heard that. Just felt a huge pit in my stomach. She said they talked about giving her either chemotherapy or radiography, but she was very upbeat about it all.

It was her way of handling it.

She said she was going to get a third opinion and ask her brother in Australia.

We didn't talk about much else, and I guess if the truth is known Misty wasn't shocked.

She'd known what it was all this time.

<u>Friday 28 to Sunday 30 September</u>
I drove down on the Friday. Misty had gotten some new toys for me from Honour.

They were really good quality bondage gear, so I got all bound up and we made a naughty video.

She knew I quite fancied the idea of being bound up, and I guess something kinky like this would take her mind off other things.

We didn't speak about the results of the biopsy then, as there was no point, and I know Misty just wanted to forget it and so did I in all truth.

Sunday morning came round too quickly, and we watched the videos we made. Misty and I got really excited, and we got intimate again before I left.

That was so real - no illusions now and I don't either of us wanted there to be!

Just two people who felt something special about each other.

It wasn't something Misty actually liked doing. She liked all the dressing up and us both being TVs.

But in the final analysis, when two people care for each other, all that gets stripped away.

Two tarts with hearts, I guess!

Misty rang me on the Monday night as she was in the car going to the Phily. I didn't ask what she was doing there.

There wasn't any need as I didn't care what she did or with whom.

She was really cheery. She said she'd been to see the nutritionist. The nutritionist had gone through the treatment, and the consultant had told her she'd need a stomach tube but she could still eat as normal.

It was just a precaution, and she might not need to use it after all.

Wednesday 3 October
I got home late because of traffic hold-ups. Misty rang me about seven thirty to say she wouldn't be online that night. She sounded really down. I knew she'd been drinking heavily and could tell she was stoned out of her mind.

She'd been to the consultant again, and the consultant had now confirmed her worst fears!

She'd always had this third option in the back of her mind and thought there was another way out if things got really sticky.

A last resort she could deal with herself if things got that far!

She thought she could leave it and still have a few years left. Well, that's what she hoped but the consultant didn't pull any punches.

She told her there was no third option!

She was told she needed to act quickly. If she left it there was no guarantee of what could happen. It could come slowly or very quickly.

Either way, it would be an awful way to die!

The only option was to go for the radiotherapy as soon as she could.

Said she was off to bed early.

Physically she was okay, but the strain was beginning to get to her mentally, and there was nothing I could do. God I missed her so much.

I knew I couldn't see her at the weekend as it was my son's birthday, but I hoped I could the next weekend.

I knew everything would change now forever.

Neither of us mentioned what would happen if the radiotherapy didn't work. I knew that the weekend could be my last time of seeing her for a while.

But it wasn't terminal - it could still be okay!

<u>Friday 13 to Sunday 15 October</u>
I went down on the Friday, had a meal, and got changed.

Misty seemed very tired, and things were starting to really get to her, so she didn't change.

She was fine at hiding things on the phone and on Yahoo!.

Close up it was different.

We still had a nice evening, and I gave her a good cuddle, which I think she really needed.

Frankie couldn't come on the Saturday, so we looked to see who else there was and found a gurl from Portugal, Estelle, who was over in London.

We both got dressed and arranged for her to come over, but in the end she didn't turn up.

We wasted most of the night waiting for her.

It was a good job she didn't come, as we later found out she was a hairy gurl and most of it seemed in her mind.

All fantasy as it is with so many TVs!

<u>Wednesday 18 October</u>
We spoke on the Monday and Wednesday, and Misty had been off to see the speech therapist.

She seemed very low and didn't want to talk about things.

She felt so distant now.

I always knew things would get difficult for us, but it felt like it was the beginning of the end for us now in many ways.

<u>Saturday 20 to Sunday 21 October</u>
I went down on the Saturday, and we had a magic time.

It was just like the old times, all over again.

We made another video, and Misty did something to me which she never had before. She was in total control of me in all ways. Let's just say I played no part in it!

That was magic!

I cuddled her, knowing there wouldn't be many more nights like this. Each one was a bonus!

Sunday morning came round again too soon and it was time for me to leave again.

<u>Monday 22 October</u>
I didn't talk to Misty on Monday night, as I knew she was off to the Phily.

She met Tina, Jackie, and Jenny who also knew Frankie. Jackie told her about Estelle, so it was a good job she cancelled with us. Jackie had entertained her and told Misty it was a complete waste of time. Fantasy as I said before.

<u>Wednesday 24 October</u>
We talked in the evening after she'd been to see the doctor and the speech therapist.

She was very stoned and very down and said she needed to sort out things for the next few weeks.

Said she wanted to organise a party on the seventh of November.

We joked about it, and she called it the last supper.

She said she needed all her disciples round her and called it the:

"Sermon on the Mount – not explaining what she meant!"

I really wasn't sure she'd make it that far, as everything now seemed imminent. I told her how much I loved her and I really did, in all truth.

I drove down on the Friday straight from work, feeling absolutely shattered.

Misty was already changed. I had a few drinks and supper before going for a bath and relaxing and getting dressed late.

We only stayed up for a couple of hours, and then we both crashed out and had a good night's sleep.

Misty hadn't been sleeping well recently, so I was glad she had a good night as well.

On Saturday we went to Tesco, and for a change I didn't have a sleep in the afternoon. We had a look on Yahoo! to see who else might be about and spoke to Tammy on the phone.

She was going to come over, but it just didn't sound at all right. Sometimes you know. Tammy wanted us to take her shopping which is always a bit of a clue, so in the end we were glad when she didn't comfirm she was coming.

Bit of a dreamer!

On Saturday night we both got dressed. Misty had me tied up in chains, and then she did what she'd done the other night.

LOL - bliss!

Misty had a lot to drink that night and wasn't really in the mood to be excited herself.

We sat and chatted and just cuddled and afterwards the subject moved back towards medical matters.

Misty got quite depressed and asked me if I would come and visit her if she needed me once the treatment had started.

There was never any need to ask.

I had told her ages ago I would, but being the Leo she was, she'd came over with all this bravado and said it wouldn't be necessary.

I was starting to hurt a bit inside now but kept it to myself.

Something bad was round the corner, and God knows what Misty must have felt inside.

I loved her a lot, but was sure she knew that.

We went to bed that night at about one o'clock. Eddy came up and perched on the pillows, and we just held hands that night.

I lay there thinking I was useless in all this and just wanted to cry.

There was nothing I could say or do to change things now. The demons of cancer had got her now.

<u>Tuesday 30 October</u>
I spoke to Misty on Yahoo! at about nine fifteen. She mentioned she'd had two appointments at University College Hospital that day.

The detail was frightening. The consultant told her she'd have to have a stomach tube fitted before she started the treatment, as it would be awkward to do it partway through. Would be too painful then.

She also asked about her business and what cover she had. Basically she said there could be times when she wouldn't be able to work or even feel like going in.

Although it wasn't terminal at this stage, they said there was a 75 percent chance of the treatment succeeding. Even if it clear up there always the chances of a secondary a few years later.

Neither of us mentioned what would happen if she wasn't in the lucky percentage.

As part of all the treatment she had to get all her teeth fixed before the radiotherapy could start and have a mask fitted to keep her head in one position on the table.

She made a joke about that. The man in the iron mask became the slut in the iron mask. Also, she wanted me to back her up over the driving licence if they ever needed to call a witness.

Joked about dress I should wear to court - LOL!

<u>Thursday 1 November</u>
Misty texted me at about three thirty to say the weekend was off but she'd talk to me on Yahoo! and explain it.

I got another text as I drove home telling me to disregard the last message.

All I could think was that she must have a dentist's appointment on Saturday, which had now been cancelled.

I got home and spoke to her on Yahoo! at about half eight. She said she needed some solitude and had some things to sort out.

I said I understood it, which I did.

I knew this was coming, but in my heart of hearts I didn't think it would come so soon.

She was starting to withdraw into herself.

All I really wanted was to see her.

Time seemed to have run out for both of us.

I felt like crying a lot, and I did.

<u>Saturday 3 November</u>

I spoke to Misty, who said she was off to see some friends that night.

Think she said she was going to see Chelsea. Said she'd been busy all day, and she seemed quite happy.

I knew I couldn't speak to her that night, so I sent her an email with some of my thoughts:

Hi Sexy

Hope you slept well with Eddy

Lucky pussyXXXXXXXX - (that's pussy not pussie!!!!)

Anyway, this is all drivel and goatish, and I only got off the line 2 mins ago but felt I had to tell you a few things.

If I had a choice of things to do now I'd be dressed with you - as you know. But knowing you wanted to go to bed, you know what I'd really love to do - to snuggle up beside you and while you lay there in bed to..

But then again if you really just wanted a loving cuddle, I'd be there for you stroking your wonderful back. Mmmmmmmmmmmmmm

(Yes, I know, it was just the way I felt at the time - LOL!)

Just want you to feel totally safe with me, hun, as I hope you do, sweetheart.

Well, actually, this isn't very startling, hun - It's very, very simple.

You mean the world to me in every way, either as Michelle or as M—

I never strung you any lines - Well, I did once, babe, and that was at your party. Just wanted your approval, so I did throw myself about, but inside it was different. That cut me up inside something awful, as I just wanted you!!!!

Not a problem now, as I know how you feel, hun, and still just want to play with other nice girls like Frankie or whoever you invite.

Anyway, the real point of all this rubbish is something you said this week and something I mentioned ages ago. I know things will be very hard, and you'll switch right off sex and dressing and everything else, and probably even someone who reminds you of it -like Manders!!!!

When that happens just remind yourself that you have a very close friend and hopefully a very caring lover who needs to be with you and take care of you.

I want to do it, hun - please call on me, babe.

So much love

Manders XXXXXXXXXXXXXXXXXXXXXXXXXXXXX
XXXXXXXXXX

<u>Sunday 4 November</u>
I left a message on Yahoo!, but then she sent me a text saying she'd gone to bed as she had an awful migraine.

<u>Monday 5 November</u>
Misty texted me to say she'd sent a reply to my mail on Saturday:

Sweetie…

Wanted to reply to your mail for more than one reason as follows, hun…

Understand totally what you said to me, and, as Manders or B.., you really are a true friend, lover, and even little brother, as well as little sister.

You are genuine, sincere, loving, and, regardless of what all this impending crap does to me, I will need all these to give me strength to get through the bad period, hun.

I just don't know what to expect and never have I felt so scared and alone as at this point.

Love and sex with you, darling, is fantastic, probably because you share many of my fetishes and fantasies, and I do live for the weekends when we are together.

As far as playing with others is concerned, I think we also share similar views regarding who we like and who we don't, and that has no bearing on my love for you… I do hope you accept my flirtatious nature and my extrovert tendencies… part of the deal when you fall for a lioness…

hee hee... or even a leopardess... we don't change our spots, hunny.

I did something which was very stupid last Saturday night, which I must confess to you, before you learn about it from other sources, and I am really sorry.

After I spoke to you while driving into town to meet my friends, I asked myself "Do I really want to do this?" ...decided I didn't, drove back home, got made up and dressed, and headed off to the Phily, had a small dinner.

Then caught up with Jackie, Jouiselle, and a cute little RG named Pixie from the South Coast.

When the Phily closed we went back to Jouiselle's for coffee, liqueurs, and had a bit of a play... nothing heavy. Nice evening, but felt awful yesterday from lack of sleep, migraine, and also wanting to tell you about it, coz I felt I had betrayed you... crazy, but true.

O... No... I didn't fuck anyone - as you know I'm incapable of this unless I really fancy the person... it was a little harmless fun only.

I will talk to you on phone tonight, sweetie.

Do hope you can treat this as a little misdemeanour... nothing more.

All my love.

Misty

Well, I have to be honest and say that it was all a bit of a shock to the system, but then I knew Misty would be all over the shop at some stage.

I spoke to Misty in the evening on the phone.

She said she still loved me and that leopards don't change their spots. I knew both of those were true, and besides which, I loved her so much.

She asked me if I was still her gurl, and I said of course I was.

There was never any doubt on that, and all I wanted was to see her again and cuddle her.

Holding her made everything better, and she knew I'd forgive her of anything right now.

Tuesday 6 November
I spoke to Misty on Yahoo!. She'd been invited as a model on a fashion show, but she decided not to go. We had a good chat, and I arranged to go down on Friday.

She told me that she'd gotten really pissed last Saturday. She got back very late, at four in the morning, and watched our videos while she had a large whisky. It made me feel a lot better as there was something special on them. Okay so they were blue, but the expression on our faces was real. You can't fake those feelings.

<u>Friday 9 to Sunday 11 November</u>
I went down on the Friday, got there at about seven thirty, and had dinner and got dressed. We sat and chatted for a while and then played a bit till about one.

We got intimate and indulged in one of Misty's fetishes.

A foot thing!

We'd arranged to have a small party on Saturday, so we went to Tesco to get some supplies. Misty made some Burmese curry, and Frankie and the other Misty came.

The other Misty turned up and looked like really crap, and I couldn't see what my Misty had seen in her.

Well, I guess I did, as I think she came along at a point in Misty's life when she was quite vulnerable and lonely. Shortly after she had split from her ex-wife.

I remember Misty saying she bought the other Misty two cars and paid for her to get new teeth, which she had lost from her constant use of drugs.

Anyway, she never stopped talking, and I found her very gauche and to be honest downright rude. She kept rattling on about politics in order to try to impress everyone, but no one took much notice of her.

While she was there she ordered some drugs, and when the dealer arrived she didn't have the money to pay for them, so my Misty did.

That really annoyed her, as it was a very cheap trick to play.

Was really funny when the dealer turned up, as I think he got an eyeful of the four of us sitting round the kitchen table.

The other Misty kept trying to goad me into taking some drugs, and I got very annoyed when she kept asking why I wouldn't and what I was afraid of.

She was a complete pratt!

Anyway, the night was a complete disaster. Frankie left at three and Misty at four.

My Misty said she realised that she couldn't wind the clock back with the other Misty, and I think she wondered what she had seen in her.

It was history, and she wasn't the way she'd remembered her.

She was still just a taker for herself.

Saturday 17 and Sunday 18 November

Misty went to the dentist on Friday. It was only an initial check, so I went down on the Saturday.

We both got dressed, and I got a bit pissed and ended up falling asleep, which was a real waste. But I don't think Misty minded too much, as she didn't seem to have the energy she previously had.

Things were starting to get to her. She talked about us going on holiday to Jamaica after the treatment had finished. Think that was wishful thinking.

I reminded her about the tattoo which we'd been talking about for ages.

We decided I'd get one on of my arse cheeks. It was going to be a red rose with a little label on it that said Misty. Would make us both feel like I belonged to her.

LOL!

Monday 19 November

Misty rang me in the evening. She was at the Phily for a meal and to meet a few people.

She seemed to be back to her normal self and said she wanted to see me on Friday.

Life went on!

<u>Saturday 24 November</u>

I didn't go down on the Friday, as she went to the dentist, so we arranged for Saturday.

Misty sent me a text message which said,

"You are the only thing that makes life worth living at the moment."

That made me cry!

I went down on the Saturday, but I felt a bit unwell, so didn't feel like playing much. Misty mentioned that she'd been chatting to Monika and she might be coming over.

I wasn't too keen on the idea, as I just had a feeling about her.

In the end she couldn't come, as she couldn't get the drugs she said she needed, so I guess I made the right decision. Think she was into some hard stuff and I could never understand why some people needed drugs to turn them on. It never seemed real to me.

We dressed on Saturday night, and Misty told me that the dentist was going remove all her roots. Sounded horrific, and I knew she hated going to the dentist.

Everything had to be cleaned up before any radiotherapy could commence.

Wouldn't be long before it all started.

<u>Monday 26 November</u>
Misty texted me to say she needed to speak to me at eight. Wasn't sure what that meant, but it sounded important.

She didn't ring me, so I called her.

She'd been to the dentist, who said he would take all her roots out and also an impacted wisdom tooth that had been left there for twenty years.

Then she said she needed to speak to the consultant to see if she'd need to have a general anaesthetic for that.

I could tell she was very, very down, so we didn't talk for long.

She was off to bed early - very depressed, I guess.

<u>Thursday 29 November</u>
Misty went to the dentist and had some fillings done as the start of her treatment, which included a root canal.

I didn't go down on the thirtieth as Misty was in a lot of pain, so I sent her a letter on pink notepaper with a little toe ring.

Soppy letter as follows.

Darling Misty,

Was in town yesterday and found this little ring, so I hope it arrives by Tuesday.

I was going to send you a Christmas card, but then I thought I'd send you a little note, as it seems more personal.

This is not a Dear John letter, and you should know me better than that.

In fact it's quite the opposite.

Just wanted to tell you a few things before all the rubbish you have to go through starts.

So it goes a bit like this - straight from the heart.

I love you very deeply, as I hope you already know.

I've never ever met a girl or gurl who made me feel so happy.

Whatever happens I want to be there when your new life starts.

I know that over the next few months you won't feel much like talking and will maybe draw in on yourself.

I'll wait.

A while ago you mentioned a "needs must" in terms of me meeting others, and you said it yesterday, wondering if I'd send you a Dear John letter.

It's much more of a Darling Misty letter saying how much I miss you after only one weekend.

I know you, sweetheart, and would forgive you of anything at all!

I ask for nothing back. I just want you to come through all this.

Love you so much, darling

Manders XXXXXXXXXXXXX

Misty had another appointment the next week.

Wednesday 5 December

She went back to the dentist on the fifth, and this time they took her wisdom tooth out with a local anaesthetic.

She sent me a text which said it had taken two surgeons ninety minutes to extract it.

I got home in the evening, and she'd left me a message on Yahoo! that said she was off to bed and in a lot of pain.

Misty wanted to meet on Saturday, but she was due back on Friday to have the rest of her roots out. She pretended she'd be okay.

Spoke to her on the Thursday, and she said she might cancel the Friday appointment because she was too sore.

Then she mentioned she had to have another three teeth extracted in addition to her roots.

She'd forgotten to tell me about that!

It seemed like we might meet on the Saturday after all if she was okay.

Misty rang me on the Saturday morning to say she was okay, so I went down to see her. I got there at about three in the afternoon. We sat and chatted, and she told me she had a confession to make.

She said she'd had a gurl round on the Monday and had a little play, but it ended early and the gurl left at twelve.

Guess leopards never do change their spots. Besides I could hardly blame her for making up for the time that was running out fast.

Anyway, we chatted, and the gurl wanted to come round and meet us both. She came over, and she was quite nice.

Her name was Samantha, and she was originally from South Africa.

I took her upstairs and did her makeup, and then we sat downstairs and chatted and played a bit.

As we talked afterwards Samantha let it slip that she was there till seven in the morning.

Misty and I exchanged looks. She knew I was gutted. I didn't mind her playing, but I guess it was one of those situations where she thought I wouldn't find out the full truth.

In the end I got a bit huffy and quite drunk and went to bed at two, leaving them downstairs. I couldn't sleep and made a bit of a noise upstairs and eventually came down again and just sat there till she left at six. Misty came to bed, and we ended up making love.

I asked Misty if she was falling for Samantha, who was a good looking gurl. She said no, she wouldn't fall for anyone else but me, which was all I really needed to hear.

Looking back, it was very much like our early days, with the excitement of staying up talking for ages, and I can understand why Misty needed to do that. Think she enjoyed the novelty and the chase.

Things were getting really close now. She was off all over the shop again, and I knew she'd look for any company in my absence.

Much as it hurt, I couldn't blame her.

When I got home Misty sent me a text:

Darling, you are too nice for this old tart, but I still love you more than ever. I'm depending on my little sis to help me through a difficult time, and I won't betray the love you give me. XXXXXXXXXXXXXX

I sat and cried at that and then went to bed at half past six feeling absolutely shattered.

<u>Wednesday 9 December</u>
I spoke to Misty on Yahoo! and then on the phone. She was off to see the dentist on Thursday to see if they could start removing the roots.

I wanted to see her that weekend, but I'd have to see how she was.

<u>Thursday 13 December</u>
I logged onto Chix and was contacted by Steph from Kettering who was a lovely gurl. She asked me if that was Misty in my pictures. I said yes, and she said Misty was coming to see her tonight but had cancelled it due to work.

I reacted badly, as it was just the usual chat room rubbish and I didn't really believe Misty had seriously intended to go after being at the dentist.

Anyway, feeling the way I did I stirred things up a bit and suggested Steph should text Misty and say I was up for it. Well, she must have sent the text, because Misty came onto Yahoo! at about eight thirty, and we talked for ages.

Misty was arranging things all over the shop just to feel needed, I guess.

She told me I was her gurl and that she still loved me. I guess I knew she did, and I knew that a lot of what she was doing now was because of what was coming up.

Saturday 15 December

I didn't see Misty this weekend, as I had to go Christmas shopping and sort out my house, which I hadn't touched for months.

I bought a load of presents for the relatives and posted them all off.

Misty and I spoke on the phone at the weekend. She was okay and had stayed in all weekend sorting her own house out.

Getting ready for the onslaught I guess.

Monday 17 December

Spoke to Misty in the evening and she seemed down and confused.

Told me I was putting her under pressure, which I wasn't.

Think it was all a backlash from the past few days.

It upset me a lot at the time, but I should have known it was all part and parcel of what was going on.

I sent her a mail of what I really felt, and it was true!

Another soppy mail.

Hi Babe

Just got of the phone to you and going to bed, sweetheart.

I hope you really do know how I feel in all honesty!!!!!!!!

It's not just the brilliant sex and getting dressed and all the other tranny rubbish which I love.

You infuriate the hell out of me if I'm honest.

You flirt and play like nothing on Earth, you big tart, and still I love you so much I was crying tonight, babe, because you told me I put you under pressure.

Never meant to hun - last thing on my mind, babe.

I'll be there for you as long as you want this little sub!!!!

Christmas, New Year - who cares?

All I need is the chance to cuddle you and hopefully, if you'll let me, take a little care of you over the next few months.

Couldn't in all honesty care how you're dressed or shaved or anything like that - I know how you feel inside, and that's what's important

<u>Saturday 22 to Monday 24 December</u>
I went down for the three days before Christmas, and we exchanged presents and had a lovely time together.

I bought her a leopard skin bag and some bits of cheap jewellery which I thought went well with it. Misty brought me some perfume, Midnight Poison.

We stayed in the whole time, and it was just like the early days. Like the old times all over again with the same touchy-feely stuff. I couldn't stay for Christmas Day as I had my son at home, so I drove back on Christmas Eve.

Misty was off to the Phily for Christmas dinner, so she rang me in the morning to say Merry Christmas before she set off. It was strange to think that on Christmas Day she got all dressed up and then drove across town to go there. Not your normal Christmas, I guess, but if you are a TV and alone at that time of the year, what else do you do?

I know a lot of single TVs just stay in by themselves at that time of the year and it can be very lonely when you should be with friends or family. Misty told me that she'd spent a few Christmas's alone so I was glad she was out this year.

Anyway, the gay guys were there along with a few couples (TVs with their wives). Apparently at some stage the cooker broke down, so there was a bit of panic in the kitchen.

Misty went in her leopard skin top, white trousers, and a gold jacket and took my gold bag with her.

Misty ready for Christmas dinner at the Phily

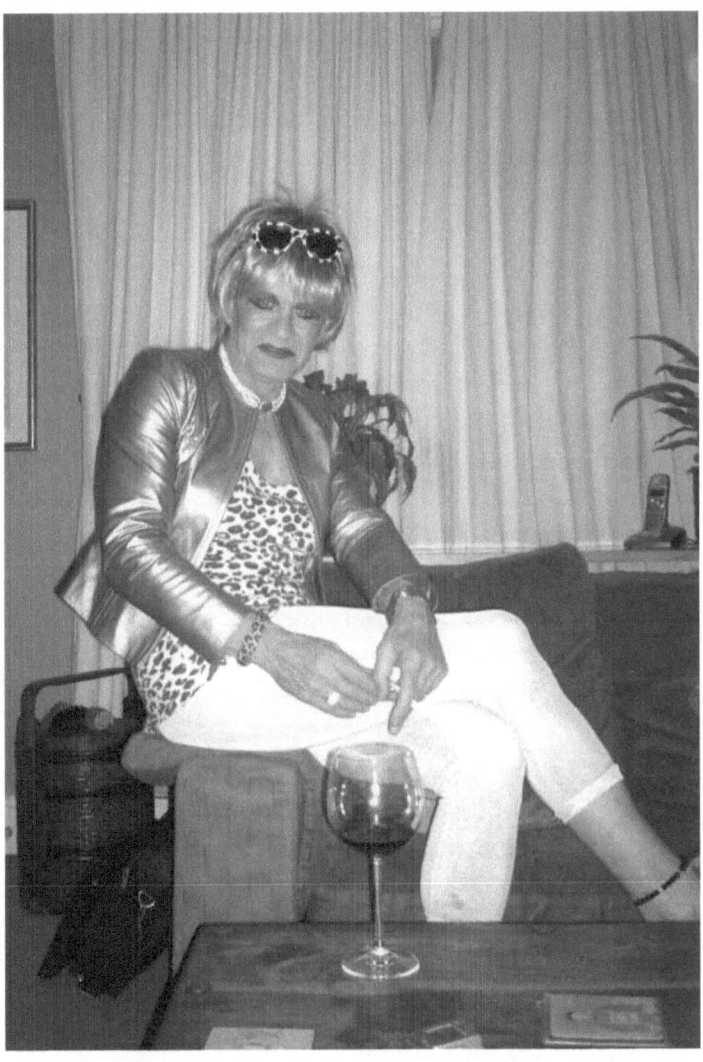

In between Christmas and the new year I had to have my car fixed, so I booked it in so they could do it on the twenty-seventh and the twenty-eighth before going back to see Misty for New Year's Eve.

I logged onto Chix on Boxing Day and suddenly got pinged by someone called Kinky Boots. He said he'd been round to Misty's on Christmas Day evening and watched us in our videos and played with her.

I got really upset and went off to the pub to get drunk and sent Misty a stroppy text. She rang me back that night and we had another heart to heart and it was okay.

Not making excuses for her, but she was there alone on what could have been her last Christmas. Apparently he had arranged to say hello to her at the Phily on Christmas Day and went back to Misty's and just had a little play.

I guess it was only sex with some admirer who dressed up in leathers, and she never normally does admirers.

I was still going on the twenty-eighth if the car was fixed.

When I think back, Misty was there totally alone at the worst time of the year, and she had no idea what was round the corner.

She knew she had so little time left and didn't know if she'd come out the other side of it.

<u>Wednesday 28 December</u>
I got the car fixed at around midday and drove off down to see Misty. My son was quite pleased to see me leave and I knew he'd be holding a party on New Years Eve. I arrived at about six o'clock.

When I got to Misty it was always the same. Any doubts I had at the other end of the phone just disappeared.

All I knew was that I wanted to be there and nothing else mattered. Had a lovely night, got dressed as normal and sat and drank some wine and cuddled a bit. We arranged to have someone over on the twenty-ninth for some entertainment.

It was an admirer who looked okay in his piccies. Misty spoke to him on the phone and said he sounded reasonable. He turned up and we chatted a bit, but Misty didn't fancy him at all and was having none of it. So he turned on me, which was quite funny.

Sensual admirer - FFS!

Some sensual lover he turned out to be! There was no finesse about it. Just a wham bang thank you, ma'am! Well, when he'd finished he was ready to go again, which I wasn't looking forward to.

He kept his socks on!

Fortunately his phone rang, and it was his son, who needed picking up, so he had to leave.

Thank God for that.

We spent the rest of the evening drinking and listening to music, curled up in each other's arms.

It was pure heaven. Misty was so easy to be around, and despite her roving eye I just loved her to death.

31 December
New Year's Eve, which was my birthday, was brilliant. Misty said she had brought me a present on eBay, which I think was a new negligee, but it hadn't arrived yet.

I didn't really care about presents and was just happy to spend the time together.

We went to the Phily in the evening but had our first lovers' tiff before we went, which was so trivial.

Some silly thing over the stereo. A lovers' tiff!

Misty was all hot and bothered before we left and even had to stand by the back door to cool down. Actually I don't think it had anything to do with the stereo. Think Misty had a flash of reality about the new year, and what might be in store for her.

She soon recovered, and the taxi arrived with the little Irish driver who came last time.

We had a real ball!

The gay guys were there, and we had a fantastic laugh with them.

There were quite a lot of gurlz we knew, and Jackie was there too. We kept getting followed by this dwarf, but eventually he settled on Jackie, who was about twice his size.

They had introduced a smoking ban, so we had to keep popping outside to light up. They had a large table out there, and everyone had left their drinks on it.

Misty was well stoned and decided she'd sit on the table after she'd fallen down the steps. The whole thing collapsed, with her sitting in the middle of it.

We left at about one, but it was five before we got to bed. We just sat at home, talking and cuddling, and if I'm honest, making love.

Neither of us could perform, but it didn't seem to matter.

Misty placed her head on my lap, and I stroked it as she dozed off.

It was a magical time.

<u>Tuesday 2 January 2008</u>
I went back to work, and Misty sent me a text which said she was lost without me.

I felt exactly the same, as I was even more in love with her now and dreaded to think what might happen.

No one knew what was round the corner.

In the evening we spoke on both Yahoo! and the phone.

I said I wasn't expecting to see her at the weekend, as she was having the last of her roots out on Friday the fifth. She was a bit shocked at this and said she'd be okay on the Saturday, but I knew she probably wouldn't be.

She'd ring me and we'd have to play it by ear.

Things were about to start soon, and I really missed her so much and just wanted to be there.

I felt like I understood a few things now after the weeks up to Christmas and the New Year.

Okay, I knew she had a roving eye, and she'd play around a bit in the next few weeks, but then she had always said she would. I couldn't blame her now.

I know if it was me I wouldn't, but then we were different people, and I guess it's a case of opposites attracting each other.

I loved her so much and felt very connected. I just wanted to do what I could to help her.

Misty said that Eddy had a cold and she was taking him to the vet.

I hope he's okay, as he's such a lovely pussy. Misty said he didn't have a bad bone in his body, which I know was right.

Really hope nothing happens to him, as it would be devastating for her.

I just hope I can see her at the weekend.

Not too much time left now.

<u>Wednesday 3 January</u>
Misty rang in the early evening.

She'd taken Eddy to the vet, and they took a sample of his blood and gave him some antibiotics.

They charged 180 pounds for that treatment, but he was worth it.

Gorgeous pussy!

The vet said he could feel Eddy's thyroid, and I didn't like the sound of that.

I hoped Eddy would be fine, as I'd hate anything to happen to him.

I went to have a bath as I was knackered and rang Misty a bit later.

She wanted me to go on Saturday, but we'd have to see how she was.

Last time I was there I took the wig home which Misty had given me.

She spotted that and joked about me going out on a needs must basis.

I said I wouldn't, and I meant it at the time.

She's the only thing that matters to me now.

I told her she was my world.

I told Misty I'd text her before her dental appointment on Friday.

Imagine having all your roots out!

<u>Friday 4 January</u>
Misty rang me at about seven in the evening. She was in a dreadful state and obviously in a lot of pain.

She said she'd had all her remaining top teeth removed and they had made her another appointment for the first of February to remove three bottom teeth.

It meant everything was on hold now in terms of her starting treatment, and it would be at least mid-February before they could commence that.

Misty said the weekend was off, which of course I knew.

<u>Saturday 5 January</u>
Misty rang me at about ten. She was still feeling very sore, which was not surprising, but she sounded a lot better.

She managed to sleep through the entire night, which was good, but woke up covered in sweat.

We talked about what we were both doing for the weekend, which in her case was not much. It was lovely to talk to her, and I have a lot admiration for the way she dealt with all the dental treatment so far.

She had a morbid fear of dentists!

<u>Sunday 6 January</u>

I spoke to her twice on the Sunday, and she was a lot better by now.

She had even managed to eat some soup.

Misty had been speaking to Carole in High Wycombe and told her we might go over together soon.

She'd said she told Carole she loved me to death, which was nice to hear.

We spoke about the stomach tube, and I asked if she'd need a general for it. She wasn't sure and said she'd need to speak to the consultant about it on Monday.

She kept talking of dying on the table when they did the tube, and I could tell she was so frightened by it all. It scared me to death as well.

Misty rang me again in the evening, and she got fully dressed, even though she was all alone.

It seemed so sad, and I wished I was there.

Seems like she's making the most of what time she has. Eddy was coughing again, which was bad news. She said we might go for an Italian on Saturday night. I had the next Friday off so planned to go down that day.

Misty rang about half eight. She'd been in touch with the consultant and told her she still had another dental appointment on the first of February.

The consultant wasn't happy about this, and she was going to get in touch with the Eastgate Dental hospital to get everything brought forward.

There was some urgency there now. Misty spoke to her ex-wife, who was also a dentist, and she said the longer they left it the smaller were the chances of success.

I really do hope they can bring it forward.

Misty wanted me to prepare some short DVD clips of all the best bits. I told her I'd do it at the weekend.

I suddenly remembered a previous conversation when we'd talked about intimate things at Christmas and Misty had said she'd thought I'd lost it all.

Well, she was right at the time because I had, but I'd come to terms with it all now.

I hadn't really lost it, and it was all there on New Year's Eve as strong as ever.

I told Misty it was all in her control!

She could switch me on and off at will, and I think she knew that.

Eddy was a lot better and hurling himself round the furniture, which was good.

I was really looking forward to seeing Misty on Friday.

God, I really hoped the tumour hasn't grown too much!!!

Misty said the consultant had talked about the tube and said she wouldn't need a general for it.

They'd sedate her heavily, so that was good news.

She said the consultant had called her when she was in town and asked her to call in.

It seemed they were getting serious about things.

Tuesday 8 January
I sat in the car at lunchtime, wrote some more of this book, and sent Misty a text saying how much I missed her.

Misty sent me one back saying I must be psychic, as she was just about to send the same message to me.

LOL!

She rang me at eight in the evening to say she was off to watch Chelsea and had been invited to the director's box. She asked me twice if I was okay.

It puzzled me a bit. It was as if she wanted to reassure me before she went out, which was nice.

I said yes, but to be honest, as much as I loved her, I suspected she was off out to play and would tell me about it later.

I wished she'd tell me there and then, as I knew it would happen. Maybe she'd tell me tomorrow when we spoke.

All I really know is that I love her a lot and don't care if she is playing with others as long as she gets better.

Wednesday 9 January
Misty rang me at quarter to eight in the evening.

I could tell by the way she was talking that she hadn't been out playing.

I knew the voice too well and could feel it.

Eddy had an overactive thyroid, but they could treat it, which was good.

That was a blessing.

There was no progress on the other fronts. No news from the consultant, but she was due for another scan next Wednesday.

Misty said we should go out on Saturday to the Phily, as it was finally confirmed it was going to close on the thirtieth of January.

That was really sad.

She said that another part of her life had been stripped away.

Friday 11 to Sunday 13 January
I went down to Misty's on the Friday and had a lovely time.

We went to the Phily for a quiet dinner on the Saturday and made a lovely video, which I posted to her when I got home on the Sunday.

When I got home Misty sent me a text which said:

"You really are my only gurl, and you know it."

I loved her a lot, but I felt a bit sad at the weekend.

Wouldn't have much time left, but the video was good.

I was back on song and as full of passion as ever!

<u>Monday 14 January</u>
Misty texted me to say she'd had her three bottom teeth out. She said she might ring later, and she did.

The anaesthetic had worn off, and she said she felt fine, which was a big relief.

She sounded very upbeat, as she'd reached the end of her dental treatment.

<u>Tuesday 15 January</u>
The video arrived and Misty texted me to say how it was. She said it was very raunchy.

I spoke Misty on Yahoo! in the evening, and she said she was off for her CT scan on the Wednesday at twelve thirty.

She also said she was off to have her mask fitted next Tuesday or Thursday.

She sounded okay, but I could tell there was something wrong in the way she wrote.

She knew we were coming near the end and the medical situation was getting serious.

It had been six months since the last scan, and I just hoped there hadn't been much growth.

Fingers crossed for that!

<u>Wednesday 16 January</u>
I texted Misty in the morning to wish her good luck, but she texted back to say the scanner was fucked so they had to rearrange things.

They kept putting stuff back.

<u>Thursday 17 January</u>
I spoke to Misty on Yahoo! in the evening.

I wasn't really in the mood for chatting, as I had a bit of trouble at work.

Misty told me she was off for her scan next Tuesday now.

She told me I was her only gurl, and I said yes.

She said at last I'd acknowledged it!

A new club called Candy Girls had opened, and she said she might go out on Friday to try it.

I asked her to text me if she did, and she said she'd call.

I was really looking forward to seeing her on Saturday.

Got to make the most of every opportunity!

<u>Saturday 19 January</u>

I went down on Saturday and arrived at about one. We spent the afternoon dressing and chatting and planned to make a video in the evening.

We took about eighteen minutes, but Misty was so tired she fell asleep for a few hours in my arms.

I had never seen her so tired, and she put her head on a cushion in my lap and dozed off. When it got to about eleven I suggested we went to bed, but Misty didn't want to.

She said it was a waste of valuable time, but eventually she agreed. She went upstairs and climbed into bed.

I locked up downstairs, which was something Misty normally did. When I got upstairs Misty had perked up a bit, and we both got undressed and made wonderful love together.

Never seen her so passionate.

I didn't fulfil myself, but it didn't matter, as Misty did. We fell asleep in each other's arms. I arranged to go next Friday, but I knew time was really running out.

Misty kept talking about the end of things, and I said it was only the end for a short while.

<u>Monday 21 January</u>

I went to work on the Monday and thought a lot about things.

I'd only stopped the one night, and Misty had said it wasn't long enough.

She was right!

It wasn't long enough, particularly in light of what was about to happen.

God, I wish I could have been there longer. I felt very on edge.

I really don't want to lose Misty now.

Spoke to Misty on the phone on the Monday evening, as I couldn't connect to the net.

The hospital had screwed up her scan again and had rearranged it for the seventh of February.

Time was slipping by, and Misty said she'd ring them back tomorrow and try and sort them out.

I kept thinking too much time had slipped by, and the longer it was the worse things could get.

FFS!

<u>Tuesday 22 January</u>
She'd been onto the hospital and now had an appointment for a mask the next Wednesday and then a scan on the Friday.

She was quite final about things now and said she had about two weekends left, so on Saturday she wanted to get a taxi to the Phily.

Time was really running out now!

Misty had been to see her solicitor and sort something out about the driving, and that would be next Wednesday as well.

She told me she'd broken her toe ring as well, which sounded like a bad omen.

I hope she'll come through it okay, but what then? I know she thinks a lot of me, but it's difficult with me being so far away. Somehow if she comes through it okay she'll go wild afterwards and spread herself around a bit. I can't blame her if she does, but I know it will hurt me a lot.

I think I ought to get ready for whatever was round the corner.

It's been lovely while it lasted, and I wouldn't trade it for anything else in the world. She brought me back to life when everything else had gone.

<u>Wednesday 23 January</u>
Misty rang at seven thirty in the evening. She was off for her appointment at nine the next morning.

I had a real shock, as I thought it was next week, but everything had been rearranged. She was going this Thursday and Friday.

Things were moving very quickly now, so I wasn't sure how much longer we'd have. I left a text message on Thursday morning to wish her luck.

<u>Friday 25 January</u>
I took the Friday off and went to the dentist and then set off to see Misty. I got there early, at about three o'clock.

She was working, didn't get back till six and was shattered, so she didn't get changed.

She just looked and sounded so tired.

I went up and got changed, and when I came back down Misty fell asleep in my arms as a bloke. We went to bed at twelve thirty, just like a normal couple.

On Saturday we decided not to go to the Phily, as Misty wanted to make some videos.
I was very glad about that, as I just wanted to spend more time with Misty.

The hospital had also brought her scan forward, so she was off for it on the following Tuesday. So she might not be able to go to the closing night of the Phily.

I was hoping I could see Misty the next weekend. I feel like time has run out, but Misty still keeps talking about the next few weeks and how she'll be okay for a while.

I'm not sure, really.

I need to get my Internet fixed and start selling our DVDs on BirchPlace just to earn a little extra to help with the petrol, which was costing me a fortune.

Misty used to pay for all my travelling, but when she started going to the dentist I told her to stop. She had enough to worry about.

I drove back on Sunday. I had just pulled off the M1 after doing about ninety and had a blow-out in a rear tyre. Guess my luck was in. I rang Misty and told her.

When I got home my son was there with his girlfriend, who was a bit of a Goth and had put black eyeliner on him.

Hope he's not going to end up like his sad old dad, but I don't think he will.

<u>Monday 28 January</u>
Misty rang me at about seven thirty to say she was off to the Phily for the last night. She said she wouldn't be playing and would be home by twelve, as she had an early appointment on Tuesday.

I just hoped she drove carefully, as I'd hate her to be stopped again.

<u>Tuesday 29 January</u>
I rang Misty at about seven in the evening as I wanted to hear how her scan went. She had it at about ten thirty and had just finished speaking to the consultant, who said it was still the same as before.

The consultant said Misty was a very lucky gurl (well, bloke, actually). There was nothing else to do now except get the stomach tube fitted on the seventh of February, which was next Thursday.

Misty told me about the Phily. She said it was a huge night and so many people turned up they had to close the front doors. They drank the bar dry and had a buffet upstairs and a cabaret with a gurl who stripped off and into drab. Frankie and Sally were there and they got together.

So that was it. It was the end of the Phily, which was sad. I really wanted to see Misty on the Friday as things were so close now.

<u>Wednesday 30 January</u>

Misty's appointment for the tube had been rearranged and was now on the next Wednesday, and then she started treatment on the Thursday.

It was all very final now, and I'd arranged to go and see her on the Friday. I needed to see her for two days.

Could be the last time for a while, but I hoped not. She was optimistic about it all and said she could still see me for a few more weeks.

<u>Friday 1 to Sunday 3 February</u>

I went down to see Misty straight from work and got there about seven fifteen.

Misty was partially dressed, so we had a drink and some dinner, and I went upstairs to have a bath and get dressed.

I felt really shattered, and in all honesty so did Misty, so she put her head on my lap and went to sleep with me cuddling her.

We went to bed at about two o'clock.

The trouble is she keeps working at the same pace, and I guess it distracts her from other problems, but it's tiring her out.

Misty had arranged for a cameraman to come over on Saturday, and he arrived at about eight thirty.

He was an estate agent who was a Sikh.

He filmed us together and then sort of just joined in.

It was just after eleven when he left. We were both shattered, but neither of us wanted to go to bed.

We just sat and cuddled, both fighting sleep.

It was so close now, and we could both feel it.

Think I ended up crying.

I tried not to, as I didn't want to burden Misty with it. I drove back on Sunday feeling a bit low about things.

Monday 4 February
Misty rang me on Monday night and said she was feeling really down and kept thinking of Wednesday.

I promised to speak to Misty on Tuesday night, as she was off to bed early and had to be there by seven thirty on Wednesday. Everything was close now. It was all very frightening.

Wish I was with Misty. I love her a lot and I'm sure she knows it.

Tuesday 5 February

I spoke to Misty in the early evening as I knew she was off to bed early. I wished her luck and tried to be cheerful but felt so sad inside. She told me she'd been in for a test with the mask.

She was a bit worried about the tube, and she spoke to her ex-wife, who said that with the sedation it would be quite a pleasant experience. I knew it wouldn't be but didn't dare say anything. Last thing she needed to hear.

Wednesday 6 February

I got up early and sent her a text at about eight in the morning. She sent me text back to say she was just sitting there waiting.

God, I hope she's okay with it. I hate to think what will happen if it's not.

Misty didn't ring all day, and I started to get really worried. It got to about seven thirty in the evening, so I sent her another text. She sent me a reply to say she was still in hospital and then rang me to say she hoped she could go home that night.

She was okay but very sore and said it had been a horrible experience. I don't think the sedation had taken full effect when they started to feed the tube down her throat and then fish it out near her belly button.

Glad she was okay!

<u>Friday 8 and Saturday 9 February</u>
I arranged to go down on Friday, as I knew it could be the final time for a while.

Following having the tube fitted Misty had two treatments on Thursday and Friday.

I went straight from work and got there just after seven. Misty wasn't dressed on the Friday but was in her kimono. She showed me her tube, which was right in the centre of her stomach, folded over and stuck to her with tape.

She said it was quite sore and she had to keep turning the tube round to make sure it didn't stick.

We went out to the kitchen, and she showed me all the medicines she'd been given.

It was a frightening array of gargles, lotions, and painkillers.

We chatted about things for a while, and about her treatment, and she said she'd turn bright red in a couple of months, as the radiotherapy would be like her getting sunburnt on her neck.

I got dressed a bit later. We just sat and cuddled and talked, and we went to bed early at about twelve.

Neither of us felt like playing that night.

We went shopping on Saturday and got some waterproof bandages she could put over the tube so she could have a shower.

She tried it later, but it still got all wet, and she needed to take of all the bandages and get it dry again.

I had a sleep on Saturday afternoon as I felt a bit rough and then got up and got dressed. Misty got dressed as well but had to be careful about not disturbing the tube.

We made a wonderful video in one take, and it didn't really need any editing. After that we had a late supper of grilled chipolatas, instant mash, and beans, which was lovely.

We went back to the sofa, and Misty put her head on my shoulder.

Over the past few weeks I'd left my bag at Misty's, as it seemed more permanent.

Tonight Misty asked me if I wanted to take it home. It was the way she asked and I knew what she meant. It was very poignant and emotional.

I said I'd take it with me, but I wish I'd left it there.

Taking it seemed such a final thing.

I got up early on Sunday and was packed and ready to leave by ten thirty.

We didn't say much to each other that morning.

Wasn't like most Sundays.

I knew I had to go before I started crying, and I didn't want Misty to have to put up with that.

She needed me to be strong.

Before I left Misty said we'd meet the following weekend, and I said okay.

It would depend on how the treatment went.

Can't believe it's all happening now and the effect I know it will have on her.

Already I miss her loads.

 I cried as I drove home.

She still keeps talking about there being a 75 percent chance of success.

Wish she wouldn't!

I know how frightened she is, but she hides it well.

<u>Monday 11 February</u>
I rang Misty in the evening. She'd been for her radio-therapy treatment, and nothing had changed except she was a little tired.

Misty said she'd ring me tomorrow night.

I feel as if she's trying to carry on as if nothing has happened or changed, but it will soon.

I know it will happen slowly but surely.

<u>Tuesday 12 February</u>
Misty sent me a text to say she was very tired and off to bed early, so I sent her a text back and said night night.

It was starting now, and the radiotherapy was just tiring her out!

<u>Wednesday 13 February</u>
I rang Misty at lunchtime just to check she was okay. She was all right but getting really tired with it all, and one of the other side effects was getting a very dry mouth.

She said she'd speak to me tonight. I told her she needn't bother if she was really tired, but she said she would. She didn't call in the evening, so I knew she'd gone to bed early.

<u>Friday 15 February</u>
I didn't bother her on the Thursday, but we spoke later on the Friday and made arrangements for me to go down on the Saturday, depending on how she felt.

I still desperately wanted to go and see her, but I doubted it would happen.

<u>Saturday 16 February</u>
Misty rang about nine thirty in the morning and said she was really zonked so the weekend was off. I guess it must have hit her overnight.

I knew this was going to be a long haul now and I wouldn't be seeing much of her until this was all over.

She seemed to be coping with the treatment okay during the week, but when it came to Friday it just hit her hard and all she could do was sleep it off.

<u>Sunday 17 February</u>
I rang her on Sunday, and she said she felt brilliant after having no treatment. She said she'd speak to me on Yahoo! in the evening, but she texted me at seven thirty to say she was going to bed.

I think she's steeling herself for what's to come. I know I'll have to see how she is next weekend, but I need to tell her that I'll be there if she needs me for shopping or whatever.

<u>Monday 18 February</u>
I wanted to text Misty but thought I'd better leave it. I spoke to her on Yahoo! in the evening.

They cancelled the treatment as the machine was broken, so she'd have to have two doses on the Wednesday.

She said she felt great and felt like taking me apart slowly.

I told her I had Friday off, so she said it could be a big weekend.

Guess that was wishful thinking on both her and my part before the double treatment.

I missed her so much, but I doubted it would happen somehow, especially after Wednesday and two treatments.

<u>Tuesday 19 February</u>
I knew Misty was going for her treatment, so I didn't expect to hear from her. I was surprised when she rang at eight thirty to say she'd been busy and was very tired again.

It was a short conversation, so I went to bed. I was thinking of sending her a text, but she rang me at quarter to eleven and left a message, apologising. There was no need for it, as I didn't expect her to call me.

<u>Wednesday 20 February</u>
I sent Misty a text on Wednesday and told her just to take care of herself and forget about me for the time being.

I wasn't being magnanimous - I meant it!

She sent me one back saying she was having two treatments today and having her lungs tested for the potential driving ban.

I knew I wouldn't hear from her tonight.

<u>Thursday 21 February</u>
Misty texted me to say she'd been too tired to talk last night but that she'd talk tonight.

I knew she'd have another treatment today and would be really tired, so I said okay, but I didn't want her to call if she was too tired.

In the end she did ring and wanted me to come down at the weekend, but we'd have to see how she was on Friday.

I didn't think it would happen, but I always lived in hope.

Tranny hope springs eternal!

I went down on the Friday as Misty said she felt fine, and I knew this could be the last weekend for a while.

She said she wanted to go out on Saturday to try Jade's new restaurant.

She went for her treatment on the Friday. As I had the day off I came down early and got there at about two.

She was out, so I let myself in, had a bath, and got dressed so I'd be ready when she came back at about five thirty.

Misty looked okay but was so tired that she didn't get dressed.

I said she'd feel better if she changed into her kimono, so she did, and then we had some dinner.

We sat and chatted on the sofa. I played with her and managed to fulfil her, which was nice.

She sat with her head on my lap for a while but so was tired she went to bed at eleven while I locked up and switched the lights off.

I even fed Eddy, so I knew it was bad.

It was only an act and in truth she was very poorly!

Things had changed a lot, and she couldn't even drink whisky, although she was okay with wine.

I couldn't cuddle her properly because of the tube, but it was so nice to sleep beside her.

I got up early on Saturday and tidied everything up and did the washing up.

Misty came downstairs a little later, and I got a shock.

She looked really really awful!

Misty hadn't slept well last night and had been up and down most of the night, which I didn't even know.

Been coughing up all sorts of gunk!

She said she needed to go shopping quickly to Tesco, but she was in a lot of pain from her throat so she took her first painkillers before we left.

Hadn't needed those before!

As we walked to the car she just took off, and I had trouble keeping up with her.

She was so distant, and her mind wasn't on what we were doing.

I remember I followed her round the supermarket and she shopped for one, and I knew this was it.

Felt like crying but held it in.

We got home and I said I really ought to go. I wanted to stay and take care of her, but I could tell she needed to get through this by herself at the moment. She agreed without any argument.

She said she was ready to go back to bed, which I guess she did as soon as I'd gone. I think this was the first time she had suffered with her throat like this, and she was frightened by it all.

I didn't bother her till she rang me on Sunday. She'd had an awful night on Saturday and kept waking up to go to the loo and cough up all this mucus.

She asked me if I found the 40 pounds in my computer bag to cover the petrol. I hadn't even looked, so I found it and told her I wished she hadn't done it. I told her there was no need for it.

Then I did cry!

She was in all that pain on Saturday and still thought about stuffing 40 pounds in my bag.

All I know is that I love her a lot and I'm so frightened something will happen.

<u>Monday 25 February</u>
I spoke to Misty in the early evening as she was off to bed early. She didn't say much except that she wasn't too good at being in permanent pain. There wasn't much I could say to that, so I just wished her a good night's sleep. That was the best she could hope for.

<u>Tuesday 26 February</u>
Misty rang me in the evening at about eight thirty. She was off to bed as soon as we finished speaking. She was halfway through her treatment and had now sorted out the medication, which meant she could cope a little and things were passable.

She'd worked out how often she needed to take the painkillers. The consultant told her the pain was normal but warned her that it would get worse towards the end. She only had three weeks to go now.

I said I had no way of contacting her if something went wrong, but she said she'd let me know somehow. I knew she couldn't, but then I remembered that a while ago she had given me her ex-wife's number.

It's going to be a long three weeks for me and even longer for Misty.

God, I miss her terribly.

<u>Wednesday 27 February</u>
Spoke to Misty in the evening on Yahoo! before she went to bed, as she was off for her review tomorrow.

The review was basically to see how she was coping with it all and included measuring things like weight and breathing. She said she'd ring me and let me know how it went.

<u>Thursday 28 February</u>
Misty went for her review.

She'd lost over a kilo and a half. They were concerned about her coughing and swallowing so were going to test all her passages, as she was taking too much down the wrong way when she swallowed.

They were also going to prescribe liquid morphine in case she needed it as the pain got worse.

The loss of weight and the morphine sounded quite frightening, but then she said she hadn't been able to eat properly for a while and when she did it was mainly soup.

They said her symptoms had come on quickly. I suggested she might need the tube sooner, but she said that the consultant had told her to leave it as long as possible.

There's less than three weeks left now!

I was just about to finish work when Misty sent me a text to say she wished I was heading for London and not for home.

So did I - LOL!

I knew she'd be off to bed early, so I caught her before she went. She was so tired and just wanted to sleep.

On Saturday she sent me another text, which said she should be putting the steaks on the barbeque before a big session of Manders.

I wish!

She was doing nothing but sleeping now at weekends.

Misty was off to get tested again on Monday to see how her passages were. They were worried she may have caught pneumonia.

Monday 3 March
Misty sent me another text when she came out of her appointment.

"How's my favourite gurl?"

She'd been for her test and said it was fine but very spooky to watch her skeleton on a television screen as she watched the blue liquid go down.

When she had the test the nurses were playing Olivia Newton-John. She told them that she used to go out with her when she was in Australia, so they all fussed round her and treated her a bit like a celebrity.

She said she'd been speaking to Suzy Dawn and had suggested that we all go and meet at BNO when she was better. They both had a fetish about feet.

I'd met Suzy a few years before in a gay pub in Cambridge, when she used to hang about with Rita Duchess. I always thought she was a bit rough, but then that was ages ago, when I'd just started out, and I was a real flossy at the time.

Misty told me I was being a silly gurl, and I agreed with her. It would be nice for us to meet together and have a little play.

We must have talked for about three quarters of an hour before Misty said she was off to bed. She'd just finished work, and I wished she'd take it easier, but it was the work which kept her going.

The worse things got the harder she worked.

It was nice to hear her so cheerful.

<u>Tuesday 4 March</u>
Misty sent me a text which said:

"Sweetie, gonna go to bed early. Bad night last night. Chat tomorrow."

It was only about seven thirty, so I guess Misty must have been really whacked and probably in pain.

Think this could be the pattern for a while. Just want her to get through it. It will soon be our anniversary in April, and I just hope she's a bit better by then and I can see her.

<u>Wednesday 5 March</u>
Misty rang at about eight fifteen. She sounded really hoarse so she couldn't talk to long, although she said her throat wasn't too sore.

She said the nights were the worst, when she had to get up the whole time. Said she'd been up eight times on the Monday night and it had just tired her out.

She'd had another bad night on Tuesday, which was the same.

She said she'd lost her sense of taste and was now surviving on nutritional milkshakes.

It was the only thing she could drink.

She had awful constipation, which was a result of the painkillers. We didn't talk of anything else.

Everything else was a distant memory.

There were only two more weeks to go now. Thursday would be her twenty-first Radiology session.

Thursday 6 March
Misty rang at about seven thirty, and she sounded really up and great. She'd gotten rid of the constipation and had a good night's sleep.

She had been for another check-up. She was okay but had lost another kilo. She said if she felt like this on Saturday she'd ask me down if I wanted to go.

The way she asked was as if I might not want to go.

Well, of course I did!

More than anything else in the world.

The court case had also been adjourned indefinitely till they checked the results of her lung test.

Misty said the court had a new solicitor who wanted to make a name for himself, so it was unlikely it would be dropped now.

Just her luck.

<u>Friday 7 to Sunday 9 March</u>
I didn't speak to Misty much over the weekend, but she rang me to say she had a bad night on Friday.

She told me she was up about ten times.

We spoke early on Sunday morning, and she'd had a good night on Saturday. She only got up three times. She had to disappear quickly as the constipation was back and was causing her severe problems.

I knew we wouldn't speak again that day, so I hoped we could speak on Monday and she'd let me know how she was.

I miss her dreadfully!

Only two weeks left to go, and hopefully I might see her in three weeks. She said it will take at least a week to recover.

<u>Monday 10 March</u>
Misty came onto Yahoo! early and said she was off to bed, as she felt she had flu and felt really debilitated.

She'd also had a bad night on Sunday.

The consultant had said her tumour was growing smaller, which was great.

Fantastic news!

She said she'd made a decision. She wanted to bring our relationship out into the open and tell the other gurlz and her family.

She said she'd tell her brother and cousin but not her mother, who was too old to understand things like that. Couldn't imagine how her mother would handle hearing about her athletic son being a drag queen.

Cricketing tart!

I said I felt chuffed about that, and she said she thought I might.

That cheered me up to no end.

Tuesday 11 March
Misty came onto Yahoo! at seven thirty and said she felt fine and had a good night's sleep on Monday.

She only had to go to the Friday after next, and she was doing well.

I still love her loads.

She seems to be cheering up as she's coming towards the end of the treatment

Only just over a week left now!

<u>Wednesday 12 March</u>

Misty was really up and cheerful. She said she might even get through this without using the tube.

We talked about the times to come when she'd recovered and things we might do together. She still wanted to go to Jamaica.

When this is over and I've seen her again, I'll have to tell her I have a few things to sort out in terms of money.

I won't tell Misty now, as it wouldn't be fair.

Misty suggested I ought to get a job down in London and live with her. I'd love to, but it wouldn't be fair on my son.

<u>Thursday 13 March</u>

She was really down and fed up. The consultant had cancelled her treatment next Friday and Monday due to it being Easter, which meant she was into the following week.

Then she had told her it would take at least a month to recover and get things back to normal. She didn't want to chat, so I said goodnight and told her how much I loved her.

Hopefully she'll be okay for our anniversary on the seventh of April. Would mean a lot to me.

<u>Friday 14 to Sunday 16 March</u>
Spoke to Misty on Friday evening but not for too long, as I knew she was in a lot of pain.

She said we needed to talk more, so I jumped to the conclusion that it was leading up to a "Dear John" conversation.

It wasn't, but she was right in what she said.

We did need to talk more about the two of us.

Spoke on Saturday and Sunday and she started talking of:

"What ifs"

I really didn't want her to go there.

She's nearly finished the treatment.

<u>Monday 17 March</u>
Misty was really up and had had about twenty minutes in the day when her voice had nearly come back to normal.

The main reason she was really up was because the consultant had arranged two extra treatments on the Wednesday and Thursday so she wouldn't have to wait till the next week.

Finished this week - brilliant!

She was talking about all the new stuff she had bought and had spent about 300 pounds in all.

I said she'd be a whole new Misty, and she said she had to keep me interested.

I told her there was no need as I loved her a lot.

She said a pro photographer had contacted her and also someone else who was a fashion importer.

Like moths to a flame, and I said I was jealous of them all.

She said I shouldn't be, as I was still the only gurl for her.

Misty mentioned meeting next Saturday and Sunday, which I'd love to do.

But she has two double treatments so we'll have to see how she is.

I don't think she'll be up to it!

I was tired so I went to bed at half nine, and she texted me to say:

"Mwahhhhhhhh!!!!"

She was like her old self - LOL!

<u>Tuesday 18 March</u>
Misty was really up again and speaking about the things we'd do in the future again.

Said her neck was very sore and burnt and sent me a piccie of it on the phone. It looked really bad.

Severe sunburn!

She really wanted to meet next weekend and dress. She told me she'd had a big fantasy about us being fulfilled at the same time, which would be lovely.

She said she wanted to do some kinky stuff and have me tied up and looking helpless.

Sounded like she was on the mend!

<u>Friday 21 March</u>
Misty rang and said her throat was really sore. She had awful constipation and was down. I hoped I'd be there on Saturday to see her, but I doubted it.

<u>Saturday 22 March</u>
Misty rang to say she couldn't make the weekend as she was a "poorly" gurl.

I miss her dreadfully!

Monday 24 March
I rang her at about two in the afternoon and she seemed okay, but it was really getting her down.

She said she'd call in the evening, but she never did.

Guess she'd gone to bed.

I really want to see her and hope it's not all getting too much for her. I won't bother her again but just let her contact me when she feels like it.

Tuesday 25 March
Misty rang about eight and sounded a lot better. She was off for something to eat and we spoke again at half eight. She seemed back to her old self.

She started telling me that she'd flirt a bit when she was back out, and that went with the territory. I was glad to hear that, as I didn't want her to end up as some old granny. I knew that meant she was on the mend.

I told her it hurt me but it also kept things exciting. I think she understood what I meant.

I still care so much for her, but I know when she's better she'll look elsewhere to make up for lost time, and I don't think it will go on between us much longer.

Was good while it lasted!

<u>Wednesday 26 March</u>
Misty rang at nine. Her throat was getting a lot better, and she could taste a few things.

She really sounded a lot better, although she was quite hoarse. She'd also been drinking a lot of prune juice, and that had sorted out the constipation.

I'm not sure about the weekend, but it would be really nice to see her again.

I know this won't last, but it would be so nice if I could get there for our anniversary.

<u>Thursday 27 March</u>
Misty had been to the clinic, and they said they were amazed at how well she'd come on.

She was talking six doses of pain killers a day when the maximum was eight so was well under the limit.

I'd have loved to see her at the weekend, but she thought it would be a disaster with the way she was. I guess I'll have to wait till the next weekend, when it's our anniversary.

She was very up and said she wanted to tear me apart very slowly!

Mmmm - that would be nice - LOL!

<u>Monday 7 April</u>

I've not written in my diary since Thursday the twenty-seventh of March. I've been missing Misty so much and spent another miserable weekend just trying to stay busy.

I took Monday off work in the vain hope that I might see her and spend a couple of days with her.

It didn't happen, and she seems to be speaking to me less now.

I was on Yahoo! and she asked me why I wasn't working.

I told her I took the day off just in case I could see her at the weekend and stay till Monday.

She understood it all.

Misty rang in the evening at about quarter to eight, just before she went off to bed. We chatted about how she was. She said she was still sleeping on and off and woke up in the mornings all covered in sweat.

Neither of us mentioned our anniversary.

So I texted her at quarter to ten before I went to bed, wishing her a happy anniversary.

I felt so miserable about all this.

Sometimes I just wished I was dead and out of all this. I hate everything as it hurts so much inside.

I really miss Misty so much!

I got a reply to my anniversary text.

Misty said she was asleep in bed and I'd beaten her to it. It might be okay, but I feel so nervous and confused about it all now.

I want it all to go away and be like it was before.

Spent a lot of time crying.

I think it will be about three weeks before I see her again. Just hope my car will last that long and I can get down there okay.

Wednesday 9 April
Misty rang at half seven and said she'd had a good night on Tuesday. She'd stopped taking the black market pills that someone from the Cricketers Club had given her and slept right through the night.

She said she felt a lot better and would let me know how it was on Thursday.

Would love to see her this weekend.

Have to wait and see.

<u>Thursday 10 April</u>
I spoke to Misty at about eight in the evening on Yahoo!.

She was just off to bed and said she'd had another bad night the previous night.

Coming off the pills hadn't made much difference, and she was back to how she was before.

She was still coughing up all this mucus at night.

I want to see her this weekend just for one more time.

I really can't afford it, but who cares.

Sometimes I just sit here at home and think my whole world is about to disappear, and I don't know what to do.

Everything scares me now - just want Misty!

I still love her so much and want to go on seeing her, but I can't afford to make it last much longer with the way money is.

Hope we'll speak again tonight.

She didn't contact me, so I guess she was off to bed early.

<u>Sunday 13 April</u>
Spoke to Misty on Friday and Saturday. She hadn't been sleeping well and went to bed early on Saturday.

She came onto Yahoo! on Sunday morning and said we should speak on the phone as it would be easier.

I wasn't sure what she meant, but it sounded serious.

Said she went to bed early on Saturday when it was still light and fell asleep. She was woken when she heard the bathroom light come on.

As I was the only person with a spare key, she half expected to see me there standing over her. But then her bedroom light went on and she saw a figure by her dressing table going through her wallet.

The figure had her back to Misty, so she sprang out of bed. Not knowing if the person was armed, she swung at the persons head and felt a cheekbone snap.

It turned out it was a young Muslim girl who was a bit stoned and probably looking for money for drugs.

The girl howled in pain and ran downstairs, back out through the kitchen window, which she'd jemmied open.

She hadn't taken anything, not even the laptop.

But as she dived out through the kitchen window she took the house and car keys with her, which Misty always kept hanging by the inside of the back door.

Misty was up most of the night. She watched her car to make sure it was still there, and then she went back to bed at eleven.

When she'd finished talking to me she was off for some breakfast.

Monday 14 April
I sent her a text on Monday morning just to see if she was okay. I got no reply, so when I was free at lunchtime I rang her.

I'd never heard her like this - she was in terrible state. She was at her wit's end with everything.

After she'd rung me she had some breakfast on Sunday and went to check the car again, and it was gone.

On Sunday afternoon she had the police and forensics round, and today she needed to get the locks changed. She said we'd speak in the evening on Yahoo!, but we didn't so I guess she was in bed.

I really hope she's okay, because this is all she needs right now.

I'm so worried about Misty now. I know it sounds selfish, but I hope it doesn't change the way she feels for me. It feels like she's drawing back on herself now, but then I guess this break-in was the last straw.

God, I love her to death and so want to see her again and have a cuddle and hold her close.

Man or woman makes no difference to me. It's the person I care for so much. It's really hurting inside now.

I know we had some great times and great sex, but I don't care about any of that now. I just want her so much, and nothing else matters anymore. Just want to know she cares a little for me and want to be swept up in her arms and sleep beside her.

Cancer does some funny things to people on both sides. I don't even feel like dressing anymore. Just want to do it for Misty.

I feel like an empty canvas once again, and every day without her is a black nothing. I want to cry all the time.

So much is happening to Misty now that in black moments I think she's shut me out.

I was another complication she doesn't need at present or maybe even in the future.

<u>Tuesday 15 April</u>
I didn't speak to Misty last night or tonight. I sent her a blank text by accident and got no reply. I feel so bad and hope it's not over.

This is really tearing me up inside.

<u>Wednesday 16 April</u>
I was so worried I rang her at eight fifteen in the morning but got no reply. It went through to her answer phone. I can hardly eat and have a huge pit in my stomach.

I got through to Misty at one o'clock, and for the first time she said she wasn't okay.

She had no idea what would happen to the car.

She'd been coughing up gunk at night and throwing up the whole time and had lost a lot of weight.

She sounded so distant!

A different gurl from the one who'd bounced into my life almost a year ago.

She sounded so down, almost like she'd given up on everything.

God, I hope she's okay and that this is temporary.

I called her at six in the evening before she went to bed. She was very down and was going to bed at seven to try to get some sleep.

Had been a rough couple of days!

She asked me if she ought to contact the DVLA about the car, as it had all the papers in it. I said she ought to rather than rely on the police.

We didn't say a lot, but she thanked me for the little present I had sent.

Little toe ring with a ladybird on it.

I found it last Saturday in Lincoln and just thought I'd post it to her hoping it would cheer her up a little.

I knew she wasn't interested in things like that, but it was nice of her to say it.

Guess it was the weight loss and the throwing up that troubled her the most.

She's off to the clinic on Thursday for a review, so hopefully she'll let me know what happens.

Just hope they've killed the tumour altogether.

I hate to think what will happen if they haven't. Don't even want to go down that route.

Sure it'll all be okay!

Samantha kept sending her texts, so Misty gave me her number and asked me to call her and explain that she wasn't taking calls at the moment.

I rang Samantha, who was at the airport waiting to catch a plane to South Africa. Both her parents had died a month apart, so she was going back for the funerals. She sounded really down as well.

I had an escort message so I responded to it. I might go and earn some money. It had been so long since anyone had touched me, and I just needed to feel someone next to me.

Could always dream it was Misty.

I'm not sure what's going to happen now. I want to see Misty so much. I keep thinking of that Pretenders song.

"Back on the chain gang," I guess!!

Love seems to have slipped out of the window.

How selfish of me!

It's been eight weeks since I last saw her and five weeks since she finished her treatment.

But she's no better now - I'm so fearful!

<u>Thursday 17 April</u>
Misty went for her check-up. She usually calls me, but she didn't, so I left her alone even though I want to ring her and find out how she is. I'm not sure about anything anymore.

She could be in a bad way or just have decided not to bother with me anymore.

She's no longer talking about me going down to see her or anything at all.

I think she's steeling herself for the final scan to see if the tumour's dead. Think she's shut herself off from everything, including me. I wanted to call her at lunchtime, but I left it.

<u>Friday 18 to Sunday 20 April</u>
I had some contact with her very briefly over the weekend. She was sleeping most of the time, so we just exchanged a few texts. I knew what was happening at the other end and didn't want to disturb her.

The next week was very much like the past few had been, and I knew she went to bed early most nights. I used to ring her at lunchtime and just waited till she was well enough to ask me down.

If she still wanted to see me!

<u>Saturday 26 April</u>
Misty rang me in the evening and seemed a lot better. She said she nearly called me and asked me to come down and stay and look after her.

God, I wish she had!

I just want to go and take care of her despite the fact that she spent most of the time sleeping. It was really good news and filled me full of hope.

My baby's on the mend - hooray!

Maybe the past few weeks were all just part of the healing process. She said she'd ring me on Sunday night, but I knew she wouldn't.

She'd be off to bed early.

I felt awful on Sunday as I just had to go and meet someone.

Just needed to be touched - only for sex!

It was only an admirer from Derby, and to be honest I might as well not have bothered.

I closed my eyes and thought of Misty!

Could always dream it was her.

<u>Tuesday 22 April</u>
I haven't spoken to Misty since Sunday night, and I really need to talk to her and just see if she'd okay.

I really am missing her loads!

I drove home from work on Tuesday, and rang her as I was driving, and got through to her at six. I pulled over so we could talk properly. She sounded really awful and was short of breath.

I said something really stupid like, "Have you been running or walking quickly?" as I'd never heard her like this before.

Misty asked me if I'd go down and nurse her at the weekend, despite how unpleasant it could be.

Then she said:

"I'm not getting better, and I won't now."

I said, "You will, sweetheart" and just thought she'd said it because she was feeling really down.

She had no need to ask me, as I really wanted to see her. I said yes and booked the Friday off so I could be with her.

She texted me in the evening and said:

"You really are a true friend."

<u>Wednesday 23 April</u>
I didn't speak to Misty but had a chat on the phone to Steph from Kettering who was very understanding.

I was so worried about Misty and just needed to talk to someone else and get a few things off my chest.

<u>Thursday 24 April</u>
I was going to see my gurl tomorrow after a space of nearly two months.

I was so excited!

I knew it wouldn't be very pretty but just to be there would be great. Told her ages ago that if she was really sick from it I'd look after her. I just wanted to be in the same space as her.

I loved her so much.

When I finished work I sat in the car park and rang her. Just wanted to check she was okay for me still to go. She might be better. Another voice answered the phone. Not sure if I said M— or Misty or whatever.

Just remember someone saying "I'm sorry to say it's very bad news."

M— had passed away in his sleep at home on Wednesday night.

I really don't remember anything else.

Everything froze.

I started the car and drove home like normal with the radio on. Actually, I don't think it really registered inside until I got to a supermarket car park near home and just sat.

Months ago I had persuaded Misty to give me her ex-wife's phone number and said I'd only ring it in an emergency. Had to have someone I could contact, and I know Misty spoke to her a lot.

Julie (the ex-wife) knew Misty was seeing someone but not who it was or what sort of relationship she was having.

I sat in the car park and rang her. I was quite tearful, and after I gave her my name and explained I'd been with her every weekend for the past year, she suddenly realised who I was.

She knew my surname, as Misty had told her about my father, who she knew in a professional capacity.

We must have spoken for nearly an hour. Misty had died in bed at home on Wednesday night. Just her and little Edward, who I knew was sitting on her bed as she passed away.

Julie said Misty didn't turn in for work on the Thursday, and a consultant who worked with her called the police.

They broke into the house and found her. The police surgeon rang the hospital where she'd been going as a patient and got it all wrong. He said it was terminal, which it wasn't.

Apparently she'd gone downhill suddenly and even collapsed in the local post office on the Wednesday.

Anyway, she got home and just sat in her office but was feeling so unwell she went to bed early that night. She died from lung complications brought on by her weakened state and smoking over all those years.

Julie was always afraid M— was alone, so she was pleased that he had someone to care for him, even if I was miles away.

I went down on the Friday to meet Julie at M—'s house, as she said Misty's brother might be coming over to stay, and she wanted me to clear her stuff out.

Misty's brother still knew nothing of her life.

She had been meaning to tell him but never had.

I went down in a real daze on the Friday and met Julie and cleared all Misty's stuff out.

She let me do it all, as she felt a bit strange about that side of his life.

Can't say I blame her, as I know she used to love M— a lot. It was just the sex thing that got in the way and screwed things up between them.

We were both Capricorns and had the same loyalty, but she wanted monogamy and couldn't handle it when Misty began experimenting.

In truth I couldn't either, but I loved her so much I did.

Julie couldn't touch me or give me a cuddle, but in the bedroom when we were clearing up some things I just sat on the floor and just cried and cried.

Then she gave me a big cuddle.

I think by then she knew I really loved M—, and we both cried at the thought of him and the happy times we'd both known with him.

Julie asked me if she could take Eddy, and I said of course. I couldn't bear to take him away from everything he'd known.

Went down for the funeral on the sixth of May and then for a wake at the Cricket Club off Marylebone Road.

I felt like a fish out of water seeing all M—'s cricketing mates and so-called friends. They were all old soaks with lots of money and nothing else to do.
Part of a dying breed, and I guess there'll be a few less there next year.

Julie and I had another cuddle, and I remember her saying she'd assumed the role of the grieving ex-wife with some ease. But she knew I hadn't really had the chance to grieve properly.

She was right.

I loved M— so much, but I knew that in his heart he missed Julie and his old life and house so much.

He always said he could never go back to her, but if circumstances had been different he would have.

It was only sex that got in the way.

I loved him so much that if I could have waved my magic wand and put him back in his life with Julie, for her last few months, I would have.

Misty said one of the reasons she loved me was because we shared the same fetishes.

Well, that's true, and we did have some good times. But after all the passion was gone and all the gurly crap was stripped away, we had a bit more than that.

And we both knew it!

She often said to me that most gurlz would give their back teeth for a relationship like ours, and I know I'll never find it again.

Not in this life.

The only real regret I have is that I wasn't there to cuddle her as she died and passed into a better life with no pain.

Rest in peace, sweetheart.

Lots of love
Manders XXXXXX

Misty and me in happier times

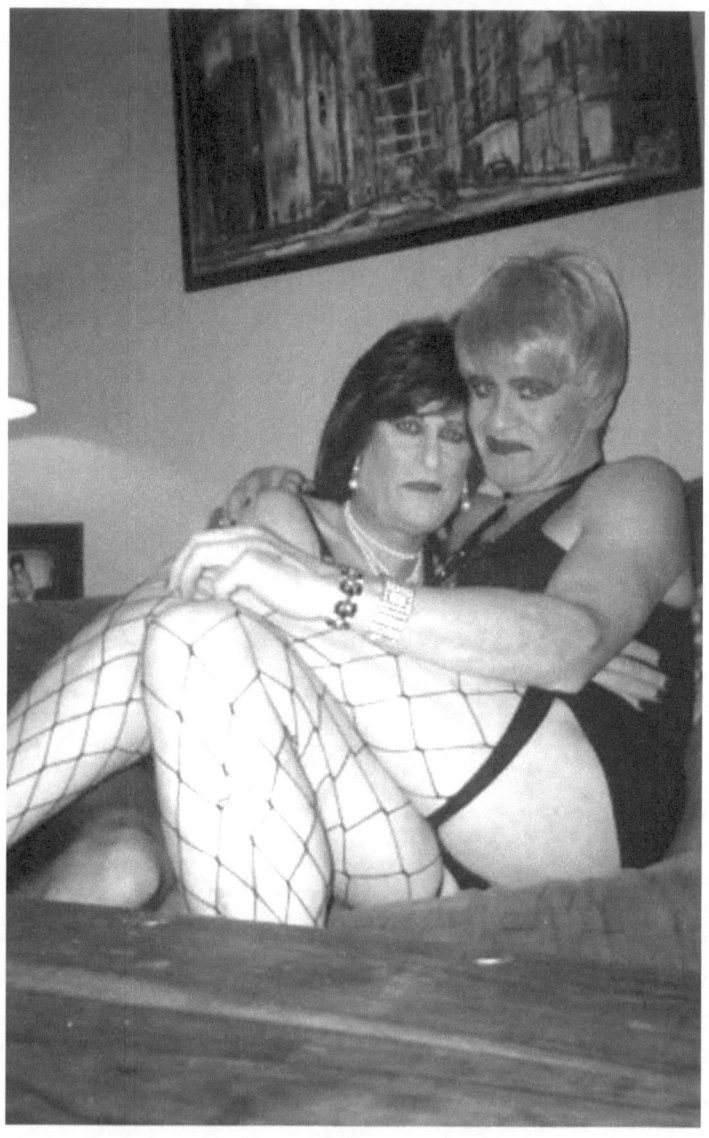